Poor Eaters

Helping Children
Who Refuse to Eat

Poor Eaters

Helping Children Who Refuse to Eat

Joel Macht, Ph.D.

Foreword by
Edward Goldson, M.D.
and
Sharon Felber Taylor, M.D.

Plenum Press • New York and London

Library of Congress Cataloging-in-Publication Data

Macht, Joel, 1938-
    Poor eaters : helping children who refuse to eat / Joel Macht ;
  foreword by Sharon Taylor and Edward Goldson.
        p.   cm.
    Includes bibliographical references.
    ISBN 0-306-43451-2
    1. Children--Nutrition--Psychological aspects.   I. Title.
  RJ206.M23   1990
  618.92'8526--dc20   89-26514
                                                                     CIP

For Don Wallin (aka Uncle Otto), who got all of this started,
and
Jack Burton, who was the first to say "Yes"

Foreword

Food refusal on the part of children has been an issue that has bothered parents and clinicians for generations. How often has one heard, "Why won't Johnny eat and gain weight?" Similarly, "Why won't he try something new without creating such a fuss?" The factors contributing to food refusal are often complicated, often difficult to understand; the answers to such frustrating questions often difficult to come by. What is clear, however, is that on occasion, children's food refusal can have many profound effects, including failure to gain weight and to thrive. It is somewhat unclear how prevalent food refusal is. We do know that approximately 1 to 5% of admissions to hospital pediatric wards are for the evaluation and treatment of failure to thrive. Food refusal as a contributing factor leading to failure to thrive, inadequate weight gain, and nutritional imbalance must be included in these figures. Food refusal, total or partial, can become an unpleasant focal point for family dynamics, assuming a disproportionate role in terms of both interactive time and energy.

General food refusal and failure to thrive as a clinical entity has been of concern to child-care providers for centuries. It was described among the poor in New York City in the 1890s, as well as in infants in foreign institutions, and then again in orphanages in the United States. Failure to thrive specifically, often presenting itself acutely, has been associated with extreme social deprivation, with underlying organic pathology, and with individual childhood characteristics and developmental stages. Conversely, food refusal in general, progressing gradually, often appears unassociated with anything out of the ordinary.

As is likely apparent, children's growth and weight gain are dependent on the amount and type of nutritional intake, how much of the nutrients they are able to absorb, and how much they lose. If the demand for nutrients exceeds the supply, the child will not gain weight. Thus, when a child refuses to eat, he may not meet his metabolic requirements and so will not gain weight. The absence of weight gain can be of concern for the premature infant as well as the full-term child who has long since taken his first step. Regarding the former infants, as our medical technology advances, we are becoming increasingly expert at guaranteeing the survival and growth of tiny, premature newborns and children who show a multitude of intestinal problems. With the more frequent use of subsidized feedings (intravenous nutritional support and specialized tube feedings), we are able to bypass temporarily many problems involving weight-related difficulties. However, the use of these subsidized feeding programs often has created its own set of problems: we have seen the rise of significant feeding behavior difficulties and food refusal based on delayed oral feedings, and alteration in the natural learning processes surrounding eating by mouth. At the same time, the full-term, normally developing child can manifest food-refusal problems that can be as disconcerting to parent and professional alike. As a result of our heightened emphasis on nutrition early in childhood with all its impact on health and development in years to come, it is becoming increasingly common for physicians and nutritionists to meet highly verbal children who have developed their own set of eating quirks that can often push parental patience to its limits. It appears that food refusal has spread its presence across many ages and social and educational boundaries.

Dr. Macht, in this delightful and informative book, has focused on the child who either refuses to eat or eats only the most limited of foods. He presents in a very forthright, practical manner an approach to addressing the problems of food refusal. Each child is different and, therefore, must be approached individually. But central to Dr. Macht's approach, and thus relevant for all food-refusal children, are the questions, "What is the meaning of the child's food-refusal behavior?" "What is the child trying to tell us through her refusal to eat?" He presents a structured, logical approach to identifying the problem and thereby treating it. Dr. Macht's evaluation and treatment of these children with eating problems have been developed through the application of child psychology techniques as well as keen insight into the triggers for the child's undesired feeding behaviors. He works closely with other members of the child's medical team; indeed, Dr. Macht emphasizes the importance of a thorough evaluation for medical or organic causes of food refusal prior to initiation of this or any feeding behavior program.

At our institution, this team approach may involve not only the child's primary physician but also may include more specific evaluation by a pediatric gastroenterologist or developmental specialist. Strict attention must be paid to the child's ability to swallow food without risk of causing choking or passage of food into the airways. Often the speech and/or occupational therapist will perform a formal evaluation of the child's swallowing mechanism utilizing radiologic techniques. Other suspected anatomical or metabolic abnormalities may require X-ray or laboratory studies. Dr. Macht always institutes his eating behavioral programs only after medical clearance from these health care providers. His success frequently hinges on the flexibility of feeding schedules often necessary in the children, with attention not only to their nutritional needs but also to their fluid requirements and to the child's individual ability to succeed at her own pace.

In this book, Dr. Macht addresses a multiplicity of issues in dealing with food refusal, including understanding and coping with avoidance behaviors, dealing with noncompliance, and, finally, trust. Ways of brainstorming problems are presented and the entire book is laced with relevant case histories. This work does not purport to provide the answers for all food-refusing children, but it serves as an excellent introduction and guide to approaching this difficult issue. The management of such children is really an art. In our experience, Dr. Macht has mastered the art, and in this provocative book he is attempting to pass on some of his knowledge. This book is well worth our attention.

Edward Goldson, M.D.
Child Developmentalist
Associate Professor
Department of Pediatrics
University of Colorado Health and Sciences Center
and The Children's Hospital
Denver, Colorado

Sharon Felber Taylor, M.D.
Pediatric Gastroenterology and Nutrition
Associate Professor
Department of Pediatrics
University of Colorado Health and Sciences Center
and The Children's Hospital
Denver, Colorado

Preface

This book was designed to serve as a reference source for parents who are experiencing difficulties with their children's eating behaviors, as well as for professionals who have assumed the responsibility for guiding those children toward more healthy eating habits.

Before looking directly at the process that will hopefully offer successful solutions to the problems you are facing, I have chosen first to discuss why something so apparently natural as a child's eating might abruptly stop or radically change. To that end, the initial chapters, in addition to offering some needed precautions, will show you how a child's total environment (including the child's unique physiology, as well as family dynamics) has the power to influence eating behaviors. The early discussion and its continuation throughout the manuscript will help you understand what factors may be responsible for the child's eating difficulties. At the same time, and very importantly, the book does not concentrate solely on the issue of speculating "why" a child's eating has become unsatisfactory. The book is highly practical. From its earliest words, it builds upon what may be responsible for the child's behavior and moves swiftly toward the major concern of dealing with helping the child eat more successfully.

Perhaps the book's most helpful component rests within its provided cases. The cases lead you through various subtleties of the process that yield alternative ways of working with your child.

As you read the cases, notice that despite the described uniqueness of each circumstance, there exist many commonalities relating to the children's behaviors, as well as the actions and interactions of their environments. These similarities have allowed me to format the book in such a fashion as to provide ideas for remediation regardless of the child's age or verbal skills.

The book's "attitude" is purposely positive. I recognize there is an excellent chance that you have experienced considerable stress associated with your child's eating behaviors. With that understanding, allow me to share the following. Eating, fortunately, is a behavior that can carry its own rewards. Children, fortunately, are adaptive individuals who can learn how to gain access to those rewards. Those two facts, and the successes that will be described, are sufficient grounds for you to allow yourself a sense of optimism.

While my name appears as author, please recognize that the present book came about as a result of many people's efforts. I would have accomplished little without the assistance, support, and brains of the nurses, physicians, and therapists at The Children's Hospital in Denver. The book would not have been as readable without the assistance, support, and brains of Plenum's Linda Greenspan Regan and my own "Schluzers." And the joy that comes from spending megahours doing precisely what you want to do would not have been possible without the beautiful children and their families. A warm hug to you all.

Joel Macht

Contents

CHAPTER ONE

Special Little Kids, Special Big Eating Problems

Parents face many perplexing difficulties as they set about to nurture and guide their newborn toward all the promises life has to offer. Most of us with children are fortunate in that the problems we encounter are quickly remediated, quickly forgotten. They are problems that occupy the smallest percentage of daily time; problems that, upon surfacing, do produce their share of anxiety and apprehension, but problems, nonetheless, that rarely record lasting impressions. Some parents, conversely, are faced with an issue often overwhelming, often unwilling to quietly slip away: they have a child who, for any number of reasons, either fails to consume enough calories and/or liquids to sustain health, eats so selectively that concerns over nutrition are constantly raised, or fights vociferously to avoid new foods or finish some of the food provided before raiding the cookie jar. Feeding, which should be a pleasant, loving interchange between parent and child, becomes a constant source of stress for both parties involved. The impressions experienced by both parent and child, fueled by daily, perhaps hourly, confrontations, can begin to weaken the strongest of family bonds.

Introduction

Over the past several years, I have worked with over 200 children designated as partial or total food refusers, many carrying the descriptive label of "failure to thrive," others simply "picky" eaters, ranging from near birth to 8 years of age and predominantly from the Denver metropolitan area. I am an educational psychologist at the University of Denver. I have served (and presently serve) as a consultant to a wide variety of educational systems, sheltered workshops, community living facilities, and hospitals that have accepted responsibility for an equally varied group of individuals. Admittedly, 4 years prior to this writing, I had little knowledge of young children who rejected food. That children refused to eat, or ate so sparingly that their lives were in danger, was foreign to me. I had worked with many very difficult children over the years, but none that persistently thrashed and threw tantrums, clenched teeth, or volitionally gagged or vomited when faced with the prospects of eating or drinking. My baptism into the world of these children came quite unexpectedly. It occurred late one spring day.

I had just completed an informal behavior management inservice to teachers and parents of handicapped children who were being assisted by a special school that was funded and staffed cooperatively by several local school districts. The small audience was gradually dispersing when a young woman approached me. I greeted her with an outstretched hand that ended hanging in midair. She had something on her mind besides a reciprocal greeting. With a look suggesting her patience had run out, that she was disappointed in my presentation, she said simply, pointedly, "You guys talk a lot, but you don't do nothing." Taken somewhat off guard, I fumbled with an apology in behalf of myself and my colleagues and asked her to describe the problem she was facing. "I have a child who won't eat," she answered dispassionately. While I do not recall my precise words, I indicated, supportively, that such was not possible. "He doesn't eat," she repeated dryly.

"Not at all?" I asked with disbelief, my eyebrows raising with the tone of my voice.

"No."

"But he must eat something," I answered naively.

"He's had a gastrostomy."

"Oh," I said, having no idea what she meant and trying desperately to etch the term in my head so I could find it in the dictionary when I returned to my office. "Does he attend this school?" I asked, pointing in the air.

"He's in the next room," she answered. I was led into a large, brightly lit classroom; the child's mother nodded in the direction of her son who was sitting in a chair looking away from us. A teacher sat in front of him with an opened picture book of animals. While she described the pictures, another professional sat directly behind the child, holding a spoon filled with pureed food. When the teacher indicated, by a slight movement of her head, that the seated child's mouth was open, the second woman brought the filled spoon from around the back of the child and, with lightning speed, shoved the utensil into his mouth. I watched the child for several minutes as he endured the feeding procedures. Sometimes he would spit the food from his mouth, sometimes thrash his arms as though fighting an invisible enemy, and sometimes swallow, reluctantly, what had suddenly found its way onto his tongue. I simply stood and stared. For a few moments I was uncharacteristically speechless. When the session ended, the child was handed the book, and the teacher made her way over to where Mom and I were standing. "How'd he do?" the mother asked.

"Fine," the teacher answered with some enthusiasm. She turned to me: "Would you like to meet him?" I nodded, still numb.

I met him, of course, but I also met, for the first time, the narrow tube that seemed to be growing from his stomach. I stared at the cylindrical, flexible pipe, quietly wondering how anyone could stuff food into its small opening. Without asking any questions, thus nakedly exposing my gross ignorance, I knew I had much homework to do. When I returned to the child's mother, I offered my assistance, somehow believing that helping a child eat shouldn't be too difficult. (I also knew I could develop a better program than what I had just witnessed.) A day was established where I would meet with this child in his home.

After spending some 4 hours spaced over a consecutive 2-day period, working with the child mostly in his home's kitchen and living room, the youngster gradually responded to what I was doing and became more receptive to the pureed food I presented him. His mother was ecstatic, sharing emotions that had remained protectively hidden just below the level of her expression. I accepted her appreciation while being thankful that she hadn't pushed me to describe precisely what I had done. In general terms, I shared some suggestions about maintaining his behavior and asked her to call me after the dinner feeding. The evening phone call indicated that the child had continued eating successfully. Toward the end of our conversation, she asked if I would be willing to meet with a few of her friends from a support group to discuss my approach. I agreed to do so, acknowledging to myself alone that I had *no* approach. A week later, I drove to the designated address and was led through the house toward a backyard where I was introduced to the woman's "few" friends. Some 40 adults were seated in a semicircle. Many held children in their laps. Other children were playing near a swing set. A few of the adults were trying to feed their very young children. I sat for a moment to catch both my breath and thoughts. A pretty, blonde-haired child, about 6 years old, strode toward me, carrying a vanilla ice-cream cone in her hand. She stared at me while quietly licking the ice cream. I gaped at the visible tube that hung from her stomach. After a few moments of silence, during which I tried to reconcile the proximity of the ice cream cone and pendulous rubber piping, I pointed toward the cylinder and politely asked her, "What's that?"

"That's my stomach tube," she replied.

"What do you do with it?" I softly questioned, as though I were still ignorant of its use.

She looked at me as if I had lived my life in a far-off cave. "That's where I eat, you silly," she replied with a roller coaster intonation that ran the length of two octaves. Then, after a sizable lick of ice cream and just before ambling away to join some of the other children, she expelled a puff of air through her nostrils as a supreme sign of exasperation. I smiled, shook my head, and knew my professional world would never be quite the same.

Based upon the number of calls and contacts I've received from outside the state of Colorado, it is evident that problems associated with feeding the young child are indeed widespread. Remediating the difficulties has drawn the attention of a wide variety of professionals, including speech and language therapists, occupational therapists, nurses, physicians, and psychologists, like myself. As most of us have discovered, each child seen has provided more ideas about how best to deal with the pressing problem of helping youngsters acquire, or once again manifest, acceptable eating behavior. To that end, I have tried to place on paper the experiences I have encountered, along with the lessons the very special children have taught me.

Reference versus Recipe

From the beginning, I must express some apprehension about sharing my observations, thoughts, and ideas about how to assist the child who is either not eating or eating insufficiently. A visit to any bookstore will verify that "How-To" manuals, covering the most diverse areas, are among the most popularly read works. Having written a few myself and having been engaged in an occasionally heated discussion about the relevance and worth of the printed material, I recognize how easy it is for suggestions to be interpreted as simple recipes for fixing inordinately complex issues. The previous subject areas that garnered my attention and writing, however, represented theoretical or practical issues that in themselves were not capable of placing anyone, including the reader, in jeopardy. The topics and subsequent interpretations and suggestions reflected positions of a practicing consultant (zealously presented I might add), but positions that regardless of the reader's adherence or opposition to were not capable of making matters worse. Such a luxury allowed for an admitted enjoyable sense of casualness as those topics were broached.

An Honest Sense of Caution

But there is nothing even remotely resembling such casualness with this present topic. Suggestions offered to remediate the difficulties associated with insufficient eating, misused or misinterpreted, can take an already fragile child and threaten his very safety. Therefore, please note that much of the following material is intended to serve as reference. It is not intended as a recipe equally effective with each individual child. *It is intended to offer ideas to consider during a planning phase, well before hands-on remediation has begun.* Additionally, it is not intended to be used without the knowledge and supervision of your family physician. In fact, you should not undertake any remediation with your child's feeding difficulties until your family physician has first been contacted.

The Child Establishes Remediation

An interesting note regarding my experiences with remediation associated with eating difficulties: Prior to meeting with the individual child, regardless of what history I have in hand, regardless of what information I have received about his present eating behavior, I never know precisely how I will approach the youngster until I have spent time with him, watching and noting many issues that I will soon share with you. Said succinctly, *it is the child who tells me what methods to use.* The child tells me which approach best suits her past history, her present experiences, and her overall uniqueness. If there is a recipe to be written, it is the child who writes and communicates it. By watching and listening carefully to what the child's behavior is "saying," a viable method to help her becomes more likely.

Don't Jump at an Idea

Because no "cookbook" is available to specify the steps we should follow to help a child willingly consume more calories or try new foods, I would urge you to take note of the following request. In conjunction with having your child evaluated by the family's physician, read the entire book before altering your present approach to feeding or initiating a new approach. It is essential that nothing different be done while you are finishing this brief book. A new program with fresh ideas and approaches, often administered in a new situation, often provided by new, *neutral* people, frequently holds the most promise for success. I will introduce and discuss at length the positive quality this concept of neutrality has regarding your remediation program. For the moment, know that you can quickly lose the advantage of neutrality if you start a new program prior to considering several essential ideas. If you eagerly jump at a presented idea because it sounds good, before hearing of associated qualifications and cautions, and you aren't lucky, you will probably find yourself and your child a step below square one.

Population to Be Addressed

It is important to note that the population of children this work addresses is limited to those youngsters who, at the time a formal remedial feeding program is to be undertaken, manifest no physical problems that might interfere with oral (known as "per oral," or "po") feeding. Eating by mouth must not produce physical discomfort for the child. Before I begin assisting a youngster, I enlist the help of the attending physicians, nurses, speech therapists, and occupational therapists to ascertain that the youngster's swallowing mechanisms and gastrointestinal tract are functioning within normal limits. A health and eating history are carefully documented to ascertain:

1. Whether the child has ever experienced choking or gagging when eating;
2. Whether the child has ever turned purple (as a result of oxygen loss) during eating;
3. Whether a suspicious number of bouts with pneumonia, sinus, or respiratory difficulties have been experienced by the youngster;
4. Whether consumed liquids have on occasion emerged through the child's nostrils; or
5. Whether extensive coughing or gagging have occurred predominantly during feeding periods.

When any of the above signs are observed, it is best to be very conservative and delay exploratory methods to help the child eat by mouth until the child's physician has had an opportunity to evaluate carefully what might be responsible for the noted actions.

Physiological or Volitional

Occasionally, a circumstance presents itself where it is difficult to know whether a child's food refusal or undesired, food-related behaviors are due to physical factors within the child or whether the youngster's behaviors have been acquired and learned as a result of everyday experiences and normal development. A child, for example, may have a history of vomiting or gagging without any accompanying physical indicators for such behaviors. The difficult, problematic question regarding etiology (cause) arises as to whether the child's behaviors are volitional (voluntary), and therefore within the child's control, or physiological (involuntary), and thus not something the child can directly govern or manage. With attending physicians, nurses, and speech and occupational therapists close at hand, and nearly always within the confines of a hospital or clinic, I work with the young food-refusal child in the hopes of providing information that will assist everyone involved in determining the extent to which the behavior is volitionally or physiologically based. Needless to say, such explorations must be carried out with great caution. Some of the information to follow will help you with such investigations. These probes, however, should not be undertaken unless medical support is available to help you in the event of unexpected difficulties.

Food Refusal and Discipline Problems

Because many food-refusal problems are directly related to parental methods of dealing with children's everyday social, interactive behaviors rather than physiological issues, a discussion of effective methods for helping children learn desired behaviors is included in Chapter 11, "Influencing a Child's Behavior." Additionally, many cases throughout the book discuss the specific problems associated with verbal children whose eating difficulties are a direct result of their present environmental dynamics, not their physiology. Frequently, a change in their parents' behavior as they relate and communicate with their child can be the best intervention for helping such children broaden their diets more willingly.

Format

The following are the major categories covered:

1. We first look at two basic principles that influence the behavior of eating regardless of a child's age. The accompanying cases show what can happen to a child's eating behavior if a problem exists with either of the two principles. Further, we see what the child's "noneating" is telling us.

The information provides the first hints toward effective remediation.

2. We then move to the chapter that explains the methods for, and importance of, the initial interview of the health care practitioner. The interview provides crucial information regarding history, present problems (and successes) associated with eating, ideas as to remediation, and, perhaps, whether any intervention should be undertaken at the present time.

3. Chapters 4 and 6 present information regarding the essential "exploration," "acquisition," and "maintenance" phases of the actual procedures to be discussed and employed. These chapters discuss the specific approaches to use to evaluate the child's behaviors, experiment with ways of helping the child move beyond his "present performance level," indicate critical pitfalls that must be avoided, demonstrate the part each adult plays in the eating process, and, finally, suggest how to help the child's successful eating behavior continue regardless of which adult has assumed responsibility for feeding.

4. Throughout the remainder of the text, we look at many special concerns that can both facilitate and impede progress toward the child's determined goals. Because nutrition is such an important part of the story we will be investigating, toward the conclusion of the book you will find an entire chapter written by a certified dietitian that offers you many ideas to consider regarding diets, foods, and nutrition. A chapter titled "Questions and Questions" is also provided. The chapter offers a brief compilation of questions that parents and professionals have asked me regarding the children, my work, and issues that are directly involved with eating.

Since it is important that once you have your physician's go-ahead you are able to replicate what we explore, I guide you, as concretely as possible, through the steps that are intended to lead to your child's successful eating. Further, I summarize critical points in end-of-chapter summaries that will key you into important issues. Additionally, you will find many cases, each clarifying certain crucial points. Immediately prior to an actual case, I ask you to pay particular attention to certain details. Such attention will help you become sensitive to various important concerns that may be germane to your personal circumstances or to those you may soon be dealing with. As cautioned earlier, please don't start anything until you've read through all the cases and methods employed and consulted with a physician.

Summary

Initially, if your child is manifesting persistent food refusal, always assume that the refusal is tied to a physiological base. Have the child evaluated immediately by a physician. If a physical problem is identified it must first be resolved before the following procedures can be initiated. Perhaps the worst we can do for our child is to ask her to eat when such behaviors produce physical discomfort. While present-day food refusal is most often unrelated to physical issues, it is always wise to assume that a child's absence of eating is telling us something about her physical system. If our assumption proves incorrect, all we have lost is a little time. In the same breath, we've gained important information, and we can comfortably begin the process that will improve the child's eating by mouth.

CHAPTER TWO

Beginning Thoughts

Often, the most obvious facts are the items many of us overlook. There exists a simple axiom that governs our eating and drinking activities, and we would be wise as we take our first step together to review its conspicuous, distinct message. Excluding unusual exceptions, we eat and drink when we are hungry and thirsty. We eat and drink because we have discovered, long before we sit at a table, say our first word, or are first placed in a high chair, that eating and drinking produce two *natural* outcomes:

1. We enjoy the tastes of whatever solids and liquids we are consuming;
2. We are able to momentarily put to rest the gnawing feelings of hunger and/or thirst.

Furthermore, once our eating and drinking come under the influence or control of these natural outcomes, we rarely require any prodding, encouraging, or promised rewards in order for the behaviors of eating and drinking to continue willingly and reliably. In a sense, the natural environment, through its physiological feedback of pleasant taste and reduction of uncomfortable hunger, takes care of the behaviors for all of us. Ordinarily, circumstances surrounding eating aren't overly complicated: when we experience hunger, we eat.

Eating in the Absence of Hunger . . . In the Presence of Pain

But what can happen to reliable eating or drinking when a state of hunger is absent? What can happen when eating and drinking, rather than producing pleasurable outcomes, generate physiological pain? A second axiom is equally evident: if eating fails to produce the above-stated natural effects, the expected, often taken for granted, outcome of normal consumption of food by mouth can rapidly give way to food refusal. The following cases will shed some light on these problems.

GEORGE JR.

If our intention is to have a child eat, it's helpful for the youngster to have a relatively empty stomach prior to mealtime. Monitoring what a child eats or drinks before sitting down at the table can become an important part of a feeding routine.

The 5-year-old understood that he was expected to come into the house when his mother first called. Prior to that notification, he could play to his heart's content; afterwards he was to wash his face and hands and sit quietly for a few minutes before dinner was served. Ordinarily a good eater, George of late had begun to complain that he wasn't hungry after taking only a few bites of food. Initially, his parents excused him from the table, not wishing to make the absence of eating an issue; it was summer, and the parents believed that the oppressive heat was no doubt responsible for their son's lack of interest in food.

What was at first a minor issue changed, however, when George began to insist upon dinner some 2 hours after his parents had finished their meal. Arguments ensued when, at dinner, the parents began to pressure their son to eat. When he would complain of not being hungry they would occasionally punish him by sending him to his room. He would cry, which would make them feel terrible. The situation had persisted close to 2 weeks when the child's mother contacted me. I visited the family's home and discovered rather quickly that the summer's heat was only indirectly related to the child's absence of interest in dinner. I watched George Jr. come happily into the house after his mother called him in from outside. He took me with him into the bathroom as he prepared to wash for dinner. As we entered the bathroom I asked him if he knew why he wasn't hungry when sitting at the dinner table. Before answering, he held up his right index finger as though requesting that I wait a moment. I watched him rapidly drink three full cups of cold water. After throwing water on his face (and all over the bathroom floor), he answered, "I don't know." He then drank a fourth glass of water. Dinner was to be served within 10 minutes. It was quite understandable why he wasn't hungry. After discussing the matter with the child and his parents, the decision was made to limit liquids prior to dinner. They were provided adequately during mealtime to be consumed along with solid food.

STEPHANIE

Note the child's reaction to being given an overabundance of food through her g-tube.

The child was 30 months old when I received a call from her speech therapist indicating that the youngster refused all "po" (eating by mouth) feedings. The child was being fed and provided liquids by way of a gastrostomy ("g-tube"). She was described to me as a "chunky" baby who, despite her eating difficulties, was healthy in every other respect. The only concern at this time was her food refusal and her accompanying vociferous efforts to avoid eating when faced with a filled spoon, cup, or bottle. As it happened, I never saw the child. Conversations with the therapist several weeks after the initial phone call disclosed the following: the child's parents had, inadvertently, been providing their child with *twice* the prescribed caloric intake through the g-tube. (Thus the child never had an opportunity to experience a state of hunger. Eating by mouth held no value for her.) When the error was discovered, the g-tube feedings were reduced by *half*, and the child rapidly became more willing to try feeding by mouth.

SARAH

Note how the child's willingness to eat by mouth seemed related to the amount of food or liquid her parents provided to her immediately prior to a feeding session.

The 16-month-old had been g-tubed for nearly 1 year due to persistent problems with weight gain and dehydration. Recent concerns expressed by the family's pediatrician resulted in the youngster being brought to the hospital for further physiological tests. After the tests failed to show any reason for the absence of weight gain, the attending physician asked me to meet with the parents and observe their child. The parents shared their concerns and frustrations over their child's unwillingness to eat and drink with any regularity, as well as their own inability to find a solution to the problems. Shortly after our conversation began, the parents produced a thick, handwritten daily log that meticulously described the child's eating habits and food intake over the past month. "Sometimes she will take 5 bites of food before stopping," the father indicated as I glanced through the provided data, "and sometimes she'll take 40 or 50 bites," he continued with a tone reflecting his dismay over the apparent unpredictable behavior.

"She'll drink with pleasure one day," the mother added, "while refusing to have anything to do with liquids the next. In fact," the woman added, "she's likely to change meal by meal." Something within the log caught my eye. "Share with me, if you would, the schedule of tube feedings," I asked. "How many times during a day do you tube feed the child?"

Somewhat embarrassed, the father began, "In truth, I don't think we're very consistent. So much depends upon how well the child ate and drank during a previous meal. Generally, however, we provide her with formula and solids through the tube every 4 hours. We try to have, maybe, five tube feedings a day."

"And the liquids?" I asked, showing them an entry in their journal pertaining to fluids.

"We usually give her several ounces of water through the tube three to five times a day," Mother responded.

"When is the water provided?" I asked, already suspecting the answer.

"In between food feedings," Father indicated.

"Most often, the child has some food or liquid in her stomach at anytime throughout the day," I said, more as a statement than a question.

"I never thought about it that way," Father said as he looked first toward his wife, then to his daughter. "Not much chance for her to experience any hunger."

"Not, at least, during most of your attempts at 'po' feeding. On those occasions when her stomach probably is empty, she seems to eat reasonably well. But when she's feeling a fullness in her stomach, either from provided solids or liquids, she doesn't appear too excited to eat," I responded.

"Then we need to figure out how to balance tube feedings with mouth feedings so our daughter will not only feel hunger, but learn that the feeling can be reduced by something she does rather than something we do," Mother expressed.

JIMMY

This case just came over the phone. I'm writing as I'm listening to the caller. The child is 19 months old. He has no siblings. He is healthy and has never had any eating problems. He is developing normally.

A few issues here. We will talk about them in detail later, but let me share them now: (1) Don't try to "force" a state of hunger without having a well thought-out plan ready—one that has been approved by an attending physician. (2) Don't be surprised if your child doesn't show any signs of hunger for some time after you have stopped providing food. Not all children operate on the same timetable; not all have the same physiological need for food. (3) Don't expect your youngster to eat what you'd prefer if he has access to what he sees as better.

For nearly 19 months, the child had been receiving all his nourishment—milk, cereal, fruits, and vegetables—through a nippled bottle. Eight days ago, the child's mother decided it was time her youngster learned to eat cereal from a bowl and drink milk from a cup: she put away the familiar bottle! She placed jars and plates of wholesome food throughout the house. The assumption was that without the bottle and its usual contents, the child would grow hungry and eat the food Mother had positioned around the house. A logical supposition. According to the therapist who called, the plan didn't work. For 2 days, the child ate nothing. He just drank water. The parent was advised to find something (anything) the child would eat by mouth. Mom found something: the child loved (and ate whenever provided) Hershey's chocolate kisses, peanut butter candies, marshmallows, and chocolate-chip cookies. For the last 6 days, the child has been provided a continuous supply of the above; the child hasn't appeared hungry for any food Mom has provided by way of plate or jar.

JESSE

Our focus now switches to a variable unrelated to a child being fed too much food, having a continuous feeling of fullness, or being given a truck load of favorite chocolates. Note how a child's eating can be influenced by a considerably different type of physiological sensation.

The 3-year-old youngster was born 4 weeks premature. In addition to subsequent visual and motor problems, Jesse acquired an undetected gastrointestinal problem that produced internal pain whenever food emptied into his stomach. For an undetermined period of time, Jesse experienced what was later speculated to be intense discomfort whenever eating. Within time, Jesse adapted to his private world's aversive feedback by steadfastly refusing to eat. Once the physiological problem was discovered and remediated, Jesse, despite the surgical procedures that removed the cause of his discomfort, continued his noneating. The child would be slightly more than 4 years old, approximately 1 year after the corrective surgery had occurred, before he would reliably, comfortably eat by mouth.

ALAN

The following three examples demonstrate how food refusal can be related more to parenting skills involving communication and discipline than to states of hunger or physiological discomfort. Note how the children's immediate environment can influence not only eating but also behaviors associated with the activity.

I heard the 4-year-old screaming as his mother spoke with me on the phone. His shrieking was so intense that I asked mother if she needed some immediate outside assistance. Calmly, she replied that her son was "fine"; that he was sitting in his chair objecting to the one small bite of french toast that she was asking him to eat. "He wants his juice," she pointed out.

"Has he ever eaten french toast before?" I inquired.

"Many times. It is among his favorites," she replied in a manner void of sarcasm.

"I take it he's no longer fond of it," I said.

"No," she answered quickly, "he really does like it. He just wants his juice. He'll be fine as soon as he gets what he wants."

"The juice."

"Yes," the woman answered.

"This may seem like a foolish question, but what do you want your son to do?"

"I ask myself that question each time we go through one of these bouts," she said, her voice suddenly a little tired. "I want him to eat the french toast. I want him to eat the little I ask him to eat. I want him to listen to me," she concluded, her voice rising with emotion. "There are times when he makes my life very difficult. He always apologizes; always says he won't misbehave any more. Then he does just that."

I closed my eyes before asking the next question. "Will you give him the juice so he will quiet down?"

"Yes," she answered. "He knows it and I know it. Each of us is exercising our independence. He's a great kid. I love him dearly. The only problem is that he's stronger than I am. I've even talked to him about this. He tells me he's stronger, that I can't make him eat anything. I think he's right," she reflected.

The child's parents and I met several times. It didn't take long to realize that the boy's eating was not the prime problem. We focused more on ways to improve communication and compliance. The child's behavior, including eating, changed quickly once the parents altered their ways of relating to their son's actions.

BIRCH

Food refusal does not always involve a battle of wills. Sometimes it occurs under the most innocent of circumstances, with only the best intentions in mind.

Despite the 2-year-old's frail appearance, he was, according to the family's pediatrician, in good health. The child's food refusal was attributed more to the youngster's small appetite than to any other variable. He would take a few ounces of formula, eat a spoonful of cereal, then call it quits. Three hours later, the child would consume about the same. I spoke at length with the child's 50-year-old grandmother. She was the youngster's primary feeder. She agreed to have the child reexamined by the pediatrician. He in turn requested further tests from a gastroenterologist. No physical problems were uncovered. I asked the woman to keep a diary that would describe exactly what transpired during a typical feeding. She was to write down precisely what she did when her grandson ate and refused to eat. Before week's end, she provided an eight-page log. After reading the description of the first few meals, it was easy to predict what transpired throughout the remaining sessions. During the first few moments of an eating session, the child would eat and/or drink an ounce or two before beginning to turn his head away from the offered spoon or bottle. Grandmother would always persist, but only briefly. The child would always begin to whimper softly. To sooth the child, the woman would play music and give the child his favorite stuffed animal. When grandmother would attempt further feedings, the child's whimpers would grow into gentle crying. At that point, the child would be immediately removed from the high chair and be carried around in grandmother's arms. Further attempts at feeding would not occur for several hours.

The woman and I reviewed the diary. I showed her that the child's eating, what little there was of it, was not providing the youngster with anything of value to him. I suggested that in addition to talking warmly with the youngster when he swallowed the food she might consider providing him with the toy and music when he ate rather than when he didn't. She and I practiced the process of showing the child that nice things can happen when food is consumed. Within 2 months, the child's eating habits improved, as did his weight.

JUSTIN

Note how food refusal can influence a child's freedom, flexibility, and health. Imagine the pressure experienced by the child's parents.

The child's mother recalled that the problem began when the boy was about 10 months old. The details were cloudy, but she remembers that he refused some solid food that she and her husband offered. Thinking little of it, the parents said fine, removed the food, and the matter was dropped. Today, the child is 6 years old. Over the years, the parents' approach to their son's refusal to try something new has never changed. If they ask him to try something and he refuses, which he always does, they, using their own words, "do not push. We have never wanted to make eating an issue." If they push a drop, the child will cry or gag. They find it difficult to tolerate either.

Despite the parents' wishes, and purely accidentally, their son's eating habits have become an issue. It first reached serious proportions when he was at a preschool day-care facility. Because of the foods the facility offered, the child often would not eat from 7 o'clock in the morning until he arrived home at 5 o'clock. He would drink a carton of milk, but nothing else would touch his lips. When his parents picked him up from school and took him home, he was frequently distraught, famished, and often nearly out of control due to his felt hunger. The day-care facility offered a wide variety of foods—cheese sandwiches, hot dogs, peanut butter and jelly sandwiches, spaghetti, chili, and the like, along with vegetables, fruits, and milk. The child would eat peanut butter sandwiches but only without jelly and only if the sandwich was made on a special type of wheat bread that was purchased from one particular food market. The day-care center used the wrong type of bread. They also didn't always have the right type of yogurt—lemon or banana. If the available foods were not exactly right, the child would not eat.

His food preferences have continued to narrow. Today, he will eat no casseroles, pastas, hot dogs, cheeses, butter, jelly, rolls,

vegetables, or potatoes. Chicken, fish, and meats are not acceptable. He will not eat eggs or pancakes, although he will eat one
type of waffle. He will eat bacon, cereal, most fruit, peanut butter,
wheat bread (from the right store), and yogurt—the right yogurt.
His parents are finding it near impossible to take him to a restaurant without packing a dinner for him. He will not go to a friend's
house unless he knows the type of snacks the friend's mother or
father will provide. Taking him on vacations, away from his kitch-
en, from his food store, has also become very difficult.

The child is bright, verbal, physically healthy, understands a
problem exists, and responds, "I don't know," when asked why he
won't try new foods. When a new food is presented to him, he will
say that he doesn't like it even though he has never tasted it. He is
beginning to sense his parents' disappointment. The parents recognize they must evaluate their views and preferences regarding
their child's eating and their reactions to his eating. What started
innocently enough at 10 months of age has mushroomed into a
problem that is influencing the entire family. They shared with me
their apprehension about setting limits regarding eating. They
have set limits with bedtime, coming in the house when called,
and other similar everyday behaviors. Decisions regarding eating,
however, are more difficult for them. I shared that the problem
with their son's eating appears to have little to do with nutrition. I
suggested that they could, if they chose, forget the entire issue and
rely on the child's environment, over a period of time, to change
his eating habits. I also suggested that if they wanted, a plan could
be developed to help their child learn to try a few new foods. The
plan would require that they look carefully at their reactions to
their son's eating behavior. They would have to select a small
amount of food they wished their child to try. They would have to
discuss with their son the need for his cooperation; they would
indicate the seriousness of their intent. They would explain that his
daily valued privileges and activities, those that had always been
available to him, would now be withheld until he tried the food
that was chosen. Presently, they are deciding whether their son's
eating behaviors are sufficiently troublesome to require a change in

their attitude and behavior. By their own admission, the decision will not be an easy one.

What do the above cases tell us? First, reliable eating and drinking will only be maintained by the natural environment if the behaviors produce the valued outcomes of pleasant taste and/or the reduction of hunger or thirst. Accidentally, we can override a sensation of hunger by providing too much food or by keeping the youngster at a constant state of fullness. Second, even if we take great care to ensure that hunger is present, our efforts to help the child learn to eat by mouth will be thwarted if the child experiences physical discomfort during or after eating. Whenever food refusal is observed, it is, again, essential to have a physician's expert skills close by. Third, the absence of eating may have little to do with physiological states or organic problems. The absence may be associated with parental actions and reactions that occur in conjunction with feeding the child. Parental discipline may be the problem. If your child is showing signs of food refusal, carefully consider the influence each of the above general areas of difficulties might be exercising. My experience suggests that food refusal, partial or total, is intimately involved with one or all of them.

The Meaning behind the Behavior

The above cases serve to alert us to something besides the influence of stomach fullness, pain, and/or the absence of hunger on eating. They show us clearly that these involved children, by way of their behavior, are telling us something important: children who stop eating, or perhaps never start, do not make such a radical choice whimsically. Their behaviors are *adaptive and purposive*: the children are attempting either to avoid something they see as unpleasant, or gain access to something they value. George, Stephanie, Sarah, Jimmy, Jesse, Alan, Birch, and Justin, as representatives of all children who fail to consume enough nourishment to maintain growth and health, are sending their parents and medical teams a clear message. "Something about this eating business isn't quite right," their behaviors proclaim. "We don't like what's happening," their food refusal declares. Their actions state: "If you want us to eat, something needs to be changed."

For those food-refusal children whose language skills have yet to develop sufficiently to allow clear communication, we must become sensitive to their nonverbal behavior in order to understand the messages behind their behavior. Our task, before we make any attempt at remediation, is to begin carefully noticing what the children are doing and to speculate on the meaning and significance of the children's adaptive, nonverbal behaviors. "What are the behaviors telling us?" we must ask ourselves. "What messages are the kids sending?" Clearly, if a child refuses foods or liquids, he is telling us something about any or all of the following:

1. The child has no physical sensation of hunger or thirst.
2. The child is experiencing physical discomfort when eating and/or drinking.
3. The child is experiencing emotional discomfort as a result of previous unpleasant associations with eating or drinking.
4. The child has learned through the experiences he has had with his primary feeders how to adaptively behave so as to receive something he wants—be it certain foods, or specific attention.
5. The child has yet to learn that eating and drinking by mouth will produce pleasant tastes and reduction of physical discomfort.
6. The child is confused as to what it means to eat as his parents might wish.
7. The child will eat sufficiently and quite comfortably for one adult but not for others.

Once we can identify which of the above situations are influencing a child's eating, we are more likely to know what must be done to help the youngster become more willing to try eating by mouth. Let me share some of my observations of the children I've

worked with regarding the above issues. I would be hard pressed
to identify any of the roughly 200 children seen whose absence of
eating, did not, in some fashion, involve one or more of the above
seven issues.

1. *Physical sensation of hunger or thirst.* Regardless of age, considerable variability existed among the children with regard to their
apparent need for food and drink. Their "methods" of eating and
drinking also varied greatly. Some of the children seemed physically satisfied after consuming only a few ounces of nourishment.
Those who ate so sparingly and who could speak most often stated
they felt no hunger. Those who could not yet speak acted as
though they were not hungry. Other children were willing to swallow surprising quantities of food and liquid given their body
weight and length or height. Some would eat sufficiently rapidly
during the early moments of a session, only to stop if the session
continued more than 10 minutes. Others would eat slowly from
the beginning but would continue eating well throughout a session
that continued beyond 30 minutes. A few would initially refuse
any food despite not having eaten or drunk for 24 hours or more,
while a scant number would eat receptively even though they had
eaten a sizable quantity of food just 30 minutes earlier. Attempts to
identify "states of hunger" were limited to observations of these
displayed eating styles rather than any physiological measures,
and the only conclusion that seems logical and sensible is that
hunger drives and thus eating styles differ markedly among children. Perhaps metabolically, physiologically, some kids experience
more hunger than others. There were occasions when some of the
children were on medications for physical problems unrelated to
eating—neurological difficulties for example. Efforts were made to
determine if the medications were affecting hunger drive, but
rarely was a definitive determination possible. Overall, grading an
individual child's physical state of hunger was left to circular spec-
ulations: if the child seemed excited about eating, she was hungry;
if she seemed nonchalant, she wasn't. Not very scientific—or accurate. More often than not, we were left with observation, speculation, and reason in order to judge a child's state of hunger.

Given our recent discussion on the advantage of having a strong hunger drive as an ally, I'm sure it is apparent that the observed variability in hunger drive produced its share of frustration and dismay. When faced, for example, with a young, augmentatively fed child whose eating by mouth seemed completely tied to an absence of hunger, all the medical team and I could do was *experiment with various levels of augmentative food intake, hoping to find an ideal level of supplemental feeding that kept the child hungry while not jeopardizing health.* Even the experimentation produced its share of amazement: many of the children seem quite unimpressed when not eating for 3 or 4 days. Some 5 days transpired before one child, age 6, weighing about 33 pounds, showed any interest in food, despite having his augmentative caloric intake reduced from 2,500 to 400 per day, which was administered in one tube feeding around midnight. His liquid regime (predominantly water) added virtually no calories to his diet. When asked to describe how he felt after not eating for several days he replied, "Not very hungry." Those of us who worked with him did not doubt his appraisal. (Parents: Such experimentation must always be done in accordance with a physician's instructions only.)

2. *Physical discomfort from eating or drinking.* Only a few of the children appeared to experience any physical discomfort from oral feeding. Jesse was one of them, and until the physical problems associated with eating were remediated, there was little I could do to advance his eating skills. Several children manifested extreme gag responses whenever food, liquid, or fingers touched their tongues, and it was necessary to gradually help them tolerate the sensation of touch prior to working on consumption of food or drink. As pointed out, *if it is discovered through examination that physical discomfort is a "natural" consequence of eating, the conditions responsible for the discomfort must be remediated before beginning a new feeding program.* Check with your pediatrician immediately if you notice that your child manifests any of the following during feeding: gagging and choking, turning blue, expelling food through nostrils, indication of stomach discomfort, arching his back as though experiencing an uncomfortable sensation within his chest,

or what appears to be persistent colic. Remember, the child's absence of eating is a message: his food refusing may be telling you that something hurts.

3. *Emotional discomfort from eating or drinking.* Perhaps as many as 95% of the children seen appeared to manifest some degree of emotional discomfort from eating or drinking when I first began working with them. Often the very sight of a spoon, the slight movement of a high chair, or the mere mention of dinner time was sufficient to send many of the youngsters into varying degrees of rage or fear. Several of the older, verbal children, when informed that it was time to eat, would immediately complain of nausea. Some would begin to gag or vomit, despite the absence of any food. Some would stamp their feet and walk from the room. The "emotional" behaviors, often reflective of previous, unsuccessful and sometimes harsh attempts at feeding, required, with the young children, an additional step ("desensitization") to the eventually developed eating program. At the same time, and very important, I noticed that many of the children exhibited behaviors that while appearing to be reflective of fear or anger (e.g., thrashing, screaming, clenching mouth shut, pushing food away) were much more likely to be learned responses acquired through interactive experiences with their parents or other primary feeders. These responses, often referred to as *avoidance responses*, were always taught unwittingly by well-meaning feeders who weren't quite sure what to do when their child began objecting to eating. (Chapter 5 covers the remediation of these learned responses.) Of all the children seen, only the very youngest, those roughly a month or less old, failed to exhibit any emotional or avoidance-type behaviors when a feeding implement (a baby bottle) was brought to their mouths. This issue of avoidance behaviors, and the need to "work through" them, represents one of the major footings upon which your treatment will be built. I would venture to say that *once I was able to effectively remediate the avoidance responses, nearly all of the children's "po" feeding improved dramatically.* Fortunately, this "working-through" process is not difficult. You will be able to replicate its components.

4. *Preference for certain foods and valued reactions.* Several of the children manifested what might be called "selective food refusal," where they were quite content to eat exclusively one item of food while rejecting nearly all others. For any number of reasons, the parents of the children had found, early on, a food the child agreed to eat, and had stayed with that food, often for many months. For one child, it was chocolate pudding supplemented with vitamins. For another, noodles and gravy, also supplemented with vitamins. Still another, I recall, would have presented no problem to his parents or family physician if he could have survived on potato chips and soda pop alone. The parents reported that efforts at broadening their children's diets always resulted in battles royal and a cessation of further parental effort. Interestingly, the children ate a sizable quantity of their preferred food. They were never hungry for anything else. On more than one occasion, I privately wondered how a child could, day in and day out, meal in and meal out, eat 6 to 8 ounces of chocolate pudding—that wasn't even homemade.

Eating only a selected food was not so much an issue for another group of youngsters. Their efforts went toward another goal: they seemed determined to do whatever was necessary to be held in their parents' arms or gain their parents' undivided attention. These children were best characterized as coming from homes where little or no attention was paid to them unless they behaved in ways that irritated their parents. In fact, the most interaction that occurred within the family centered around eating time. The children appeared to learn that when they ate quickly, quietly, and successfully, they received little in the way of recognition or affection. They also discovered, it appeared, that when they fussed with eating, they received considerable attention from their parents. While the attention was not always pleasant, at least to this observer, it was, nevertheless, attention—something the children craved. With these children, feeding was less a problem than were the family dynamics. Often with the help of the medical team's social worker and/or clinical psychologist, *the parents were assisted in looking at what they were doing and in changing their behaviors which had negative effects on their children's eating.* Once the parents altered their ways of reacting to the children's eating and noneating behaviors, the children, predictably, altered their behaviors as well. They learned that eating would produce pleasant reactions from their parents.

5. *Not having experienced pleasant tastes and/or reduction of discomfort from hunger.* Most food-refusal children, even those less than a year old, have successfully experienced different tastes of foods as well as the pleasant sensation that comes from the reduction of hunger when eating by mouth. Their acquired food refusal appears associated with variables other than not having first-hand knowledge of those natural outcomes of eating. However, a select group of children I saw had, at some point in their lives, experienced extensive, prolonged augmentative, non-"po" feeding, either by g-tube, nasal tube, or some other artificial means of gaining nourishment. Frequently, these children's eating regimes included attempts at "po" feeding, but most often the attempts had failed to show the children what it was like to experience different tastes or to no longer feel hungry. Invariably, these children had undergone extended hospitalizations, either directly due to their failure to gain weight and grow, or because of severe physical problems that had beset them often from birth. (Hospitalization can dramatically disrupt normal eating routines, producing varying degrees of food refusal.) Because of the need for extensive augmentative feeds coupled with the absence of successful "po" feeds, *the children appeared to have little understanding that eating by mouth could produce pleasant tastes and/or reduction of hunger.* In a true sense, the children had experienced little "ownership" of the eating process. They were fed according to someone else's timetable. They no doubt experienced hunger, but they did not experience any active, self-initiated process to reduce the hunger. If you recall the earlier case of "Sarah," her mother made the following comment:

> Then we need to figure out how to balance tube feedings with mouth feedings so our daughter will not only feel hunger, but learn that the feeling can be reduced by something she does rather than something we do.

Sarah's mother was correct: for her child's "po" eating to become more consistent, the youngster would need to learn that her effort, that is, swallowing food by mouth, was the action that brought about a reduction of hunger. Once that lesson was learned, the child would be in a better position to successfully and appropriately direct her own eating behavior.

Caution: Be considerate of the child's perception of being fed. Attempts at "po" feeding were often thwarted by the children because they seemed wary of having someone place something, not of their choosing, into their mouths. Again, these were children who had not experienced much success (or perhaps exposure) with "po" feeds: hunger was reduced by someone, at some point in time, in some location; all of which occurred with little participation from the child.

Sometimes we neglect to think about what it would be like to have someone—a stranger or otherwise—force, gently or also otherwise, an object into our mouths. The experience can be most unsettling. It wouldn't hurt those of us who work with these children to have someone replicate with us what we are doing with them. Try it: have someone seated in front of you or, heaven forbid, seated behind you, with hand perhaps placed on your chin or cheek thus preventing your head from turning, repeatedly shove a spoon into your mouth. It might stimulate some needed empathy. The experience can produce considerable emotional discomfort and, as you will find out, vociferous attempts at avoiding the whole mess. Under such conditions, the child is quite correct to object to our methods. Remember, the child's behavior is telling us something. In this instance, the message is most likely: change your methods; you're going too fast; you're putting too much in my mouth; you're too rough; don't railroad me; relax, be patient; Rome wasn't built in a day; time is on our side; I'll get there, eventually. The child is also telling us, Watch me, watch my behavior. I'll guide you, I'll let you know if you're moving too fast, too slow, or just right!

On the other hand, some of the children I saw, not appearing at all apprehensive, allowed a spoonful or two of food to enter their mouths but wouldn't swallow what was provided. Instead, they either spit out the food or allowed it to drool from the corners of their opened mouths. Still others "packed" the food for the longest periods of time in their cheeks and waited patiently until someone removed that which had nearly dissolved. It goes without saying, of course, that little benefit to the child occurs when food is "squirreled" in a cheek cavity. Again, such behaviors provide us with important information. Perhaps:

a. The child is afraid to swallow due to previously (or presently) experienced discomfort;
b. The child doesn't know how to swallow;
c. The child sees no reason to swallow; indeed, he may be receiving lots of attention (thus, reasons) for *not* swallowing.

Each of the above possibilities are, fortunately, reversible.

6. *Confusion*. Some of the children I worked with appeared uncertain of what their primary feeders wanted them to do. There was little consistency in the feeding programs regarding utensils to be used, whether the child was to be fed by the feeder or whether the child was expected to feed himself, how much was to be consumed, how much was to be offered, when feeding was finished, whether the child was to eat being held or being seated, and a host of other variables that ordinarily pose no problems for the child who eats comfortably and appropriately. One 12-month-old child was randomly breast-fed, bottle-fed, and cup-fed, depending mostly upon the whim of the mother. The child chose to bring order and consistency into his young life: he stopped feeding altogether. A pediatrician described the scenario as an example of "nipple confusion," a term that seemed to fit the circumstances perfectly.

It is likely that most children whose eating experiences begin and continue without major interruption quickly learn a predictable pattern involved in the activity. Such predictability no doubt helps the children develop expectations both for their parents' and their own behaviors, expectations that lead to desirable eating habits. Certainly with children whose eating experiences have seen extensive interruptions, the need for predictability takes on special prominence. As we go through the various procedural options available to us, one point should be emphasized: *the child must know what we are doing; the child must be able to predict both what we desire from her, as well as what she can expect from us.*

7. *Eating for one parent (adult), but not for any others.* Finally, a number of the children demonstrated a clear preference as to whom they would eat for. Sometimes the chosen adult would be only the mother, other times only the father. Occasionally, a maid or nanny would have little difficulty feeding the child, while neither Mom nor Dad experienced any success. Sometimes a therapist or nurse would become the chosen one; sometimes only an older sibling would make any headway. As with the selective eater, these children were not true food refusers. Indeed, they were eaters, but they were more picky about who was to do the feeding than what foods would be eaten. One of the more critical pieces of information a professional can obtain during the initial interview with a child's parents pertains to the child's willingness to eat successfully for someone (anyone). Indeed, *a child who does eat for someone, perhaps to the exclusion of everyone else, is telling us that that person's feeding method is, from the child's perspective, the preferred method.* One of our tasks is to analyze microscopically that method so as to help others replicate it. Videotaping the particulars is usually the best way to uncover which components are most successful and therefore in need of use by others.

Each of the above conditions presents us with two very important issues.

First Issue: A common eating program suitable for all noneaters is not possible, given the differences within specific cases. Each condition requires subtle and sometimes not so subtle variations before a successful program can be possible. If we return to the previously described seven points, we can see that they speak to very different issues. Any particular one, or combination of several, may require our attention and remediation. Notice again that the fact that:

Number 1. The child has no physical sensation of hunger or thirst speaks to the importance of establishing a state of hunger or thirst.

Number 2. The child is experiencing physical discomfort when eating and/or drinking speaks to the removal of any physical discomfort associated with eating.

Number 3. The child is experiencing emotional discomfort as a result of previous unpleasant associations with eating or drinking speaks to the necessity for removing existing fear and learned avoidance components that are interfering with eating.

Number 4. The child has learned how to adaptively manipulate his environment in order to receive something that at present is more valued than eating or drinking, or more valued than the food and/or drink being provided at the moment speaks primarily to the need for broadening a child's diet, as well as establishing guidelines regarding what a child must do in order to receive what he values.

Number 5. The child has yet to learn that eating and drinking by mouth will produce pleasant tastes and/or reduction of physical discomfort speaks to the need for learning (or relearning) the very basic lessons involved with tastes and hunger reduction.

Number 6. The child is confused as to what it means to eat successfully speaks to order, predictability, and consistency.

Number 7. The child will eat successfully and quite comfortably for one adult but for no one else speaks to the issue of generalization.

Since the above seven issues are so different, a common "cookbook" approach will be hard to come by, much less be effective. Inevitably, such an approach will overlook something uniquely important about the individual child and the circumstances within which he finds himself. This likelihood brings us to the second important issue.

Second Issue: A child's refusal to eat or willingness only to eat selectively, along with all manifested behaviors during feeding, regardless of their severity or annoyance, are, above anything else, *adaptive* behaviors. The behaviors are telling us something about the child's preferences, her values, her perceptions, and her acquired style of dealing with a problem that may be no more enjoyable for her than it is for us. They are behaviors that we can ill afford to ignore or overlook, for *it is from the behaviors that we can learn how best to approach the child*.

Tailoring a program to meet an individual child's needs requires information that speaks directly to the above issues. That information is best obtained through the initial interview.

The Initial Interview

The major purpose for the first, formal meeting with the child's parents or primary health care workers is to ascertain information that will help place the child's eating difficulties into perspective.

When conducting the interview, I attempt to see the child's eating behavior as it fits within the youngster's daily environment. I do not see the child isolated from his surroundings, but rather as an integral part of the encompassing environment that is influencing the eating behavior. To that end, I seek to gain information that will help me understand precisely:

1. What the child is doing;
2. How the environment is responding to the child's actions;
3. What conditions exist under which the various behaviors occur; and
4. Any unique characteristics of the child and special eating needs that must be taken into consideration, as well as other pertinent material that may lead to program ideas.

Specifically, the interview will tell me something of:

1. The physiological uniqueness of the child;
2. The types of behaviors the child manifests during feeding;
3. The cues that are surrounding him and influencing the eating behavior;
4. The internal (physiological) and external (environmental) feedback the behaviors are producing; and
5. The child's perceptions of the environment's feedback.

Each of the above factors will be an integral part of your remedial program. While all are essential, none takes precedence over the uniqueness of the individual child.

The Unique Individual

The uniqueness of a child is a given. We all know that each child carries within himself his own physiology, history regarding eating, emotional and personal characteristics, along with an infinite number of other variables that all contribute to his feeding experience. While all of these variables are investigated during the initial interview, one component stands out as being especially important. The first item on the initial interview's agenda refers to the child's state of health as it relates to eating; without exception, the child's physiology is the first component that demands our attention. I never work with a young child until he has undergone a complete medical exam to determine if there exists any contraindications to normal "po" feeding. I need to know the state of his swallowing response, his sensitivities to oral stimulation, his degree of tongue control, whether he has difficulty with lip closure, how successful he is at chewing and/or sucking, whether he's likely to gag, choke, cough excessively or aspirate, along with any number of other variables that are evaluated by physicians and therapists. Efforts toward developing an effective feeding program do not begin until the child has been given a clean bill of health regarding "po" feeds.

The Child's Behavior

Once the child is seen as physically capable of benefiting from a "po" eating program, the interview's focus changes to the child's behaviors as they pertain to eating and other activities. Questions regarding the child's actions take on paramount importance. I will need to be particularly sensitive to everything the child does before, during, and after a feeding session. There are many questions to be asked. All of them refer to the child's behaviors. What, for example, does the child do when seated in a high chair? Is she quiet, does she cry, does she struggle to get out? What happens when the bib is placed on her chest? How does she react to the spoon or bottle? Is the reaction the same whether the utensils are close to her mouth or a foot or so away? Is the reaction the same whether the spoon or bottle is empty or full? Will the child tolerate the utensils touching her lips? Cheeks? Tongue? Does she open her mouth for the spoon or bottle, or does she clench her teeth or gums? Will she open her mouth for a finger or toy or blanket? What happens when food is placed on her lips or tongue? If food is in her mouth does she close her lips and swallow? Does she allow the food to fall out of her mouth? Does she vomit or spit the food back? Does she just say no to whatever you do, or will she somewhat willingly tolerate (perhaps enjoy) or participate in a small part of the eating process? Does the child eat one food to the exclusion of all others? Does the child throw tantrums if pressure is applied to try new foods?

Know that the answer to any one of the above questions may provide the critical material upon which to build a successful program. From the beginning, then, the professional must be microscopic in his or her analysis of what the child is doing. I scrutinize and write down everything that seems the least bit important. As will be said again, the child's behavior tells us what we need to do. We must all be prepared to watch that behavior like the proverbial hawk.

Identifying Where the Child Can Succeed

There's one more issue about a child's behavior that warrants brief mentioning before moving on. Somewhat later, I list a hypothetical eating sequence that all children, to some degree, go through. Somewhere along that eating sequence, the child will demonstrate a measure of success: she's going to do exactly what the professional intends for her. While her accomplishment won't likely be all the therapist had in mind for her, she will, nevertheless, be successful at some approximation of the feeding goal. Her behavior will be right on target. Please note that I cannot overestimate the importance of identifying the point at which the child does well. We must find that smallest link in the total chain where the child experiences success. We need to build upon that link no matter how distant it may be from the goal. Therefore, as the professional scrutinizes all that the child does, he must pay particular attention to the right things the child does. That success will become the cornerstone for the next step.

Environmental Cues Guide a Child's Eating Behavior

The child's behavior, that which is right on target, as well as that which has veered slightly off center, always occurs within his environment. Said slightly differently, the behaviors associated with eating occur in the presence of *cues*: people, places, foods, spoons, cups, thoughts, feelings, and a host of other things that surround the eater (and feeder). The interview helps determine not only what the child does but, equally as important, when and under what conditions he does it.

Cues guide the child's eating behavior, as well as the way the adult feeds the youngster. Rather than "causing" anything to happen, cues "set the stage" for behavior; they influence rather than force. Cues are often referred to as "antecedents" because they come before behavior. The red traffic light, for example, sets the stage, or serves as an antecedent cue, for us to put our foot on our car's brake pedal. The light only increases the chances we will behave in such a manner. It doesn't force us to do so.

Just as the traffic light can increase the chances we will depress the brake, so too are there cues that actually increase the chances a child will eat by mouth. Similarly, as you might predict, there are cues that decrease the chances your child will swallow food. From a practical standpoint, knowing which cues help or impede eating is, obviously, very useful information. The interview helps discern which cues are allies and which ones are adversaries. Here's how cues work.

Imagine two adults, both relatively hungry, seated at a dinner table. Raw oysters on the half-shell are served. The oysters represent one set of cues. (Their appearance, texture, aroma, and temperature are specific cues.) The location, a restaurant, perhaps, represents another cue; the company seated nearby, yet another. Now to the two hungry folks. One adult, fond of the little creatures, reacts favorably, and dives into the offering. The other adult, less pleased, who finds oysters unsavory, slimy little creatures, may wish to dive under the table. If propriety prevents the latter wish from occurring, a stomach ailment (feigned, no doubt) may be proclaimed in order to avoid having to swallow the slippery delicacies. As is evident, the very sight of the food, its smell, the memories it elicits, the individuals' experiences and ultimate preferences, will set the stage for the adults' differing behaviors.

Why is the issue of cues so important to us? Children, too, use cues to determine whether they intend to "dive in" or "dive under," whether they will be receptive to provided foods, or whether they will do whatever is necessary to avoid eating. Remember, some cues actually increase the chances that a child will eat. We have to identify the cuing conditions under which eating does, as well as does not, take place. When, for example, a child eats for one adult but not for another, she is telling us that there exists an important difference between the two adults. Adult A presents different cues than adult B. The child has learned that individual A does something different from individual B. The child likes something about A that apparently B does not provide. Is such an observation important? Understatedly, "you bet." We must find out the differences between the two: one feeder has figured out what to do, while the other hasn't. Because the child has shown us that A somehow is "better" (read more effective) than B, she has also shown us where to look to find the correct remedial approach. Children, fortunately, do that: they tell us how to help them.

Different foods also provide cues that often impact a child's behavior. Try the following exercise. A child willingly eats chocolate pudding. Place a bowl of chicken-flavored rice (or nearly anything else) in front of him and he screams, gags, or says, "I won't eat it." Take a second to identify which cues may be influencing the child's eating behavior. We know he eats chocolate pudding. What associating cues may set the stage for the child to successfully swallow the pudding? (This happens to be much more complicated than it may first appear. Try it, nevertheless. There's a very important reason for doing so.) I can think of at least five cues: color, taste, texture, aroma, familiarity. Why such a big deal? Suppose texture is the *key* cue—the one critical cue the child uses to determine whether he will or will not swallow. Could you figure out a way to use that cue to broaden the child's diet? How about banana pudding as a possibility? Same texture as the desired chocolate pudding, thus from that standpoint at least, banana pudding provides one similar cue. Suppose instead of texture, the key cue was taste? The kid loves the taste of chocolate. What form or shape it takes is less relevant. Any ideas how you might alter his diet? How about pancakes or mashed potatoes drowned in chocolate syrup? It's a possibility. The important point regarding this exercise is that the child will often tell us what cues have become positively associated with foods being eaten. For a particular child, a food's appearance or its aroma might be the cues we need to build upon. How nice it would be to help a child eat better by simply making his or her food more attractive.

Let's change directions from foods and return to people once more. There's something very important about this cuing business as it relates to adult feeders. Think again of our individual A and individual B mentioned earlier. Remember, the child ate fine in the presence of one adult but not in the presence of the other. Cue: Different people.

CARLY

Try figuring out the differences in cues that might exist (and thus be perceived by a child) between different people. The following story contains three real people. What happened was precisely as described. Speculate on what cuing differences might have been responsible for the child's differential behavior. Think of how essential, not to mention helpful, it would be to determine which of the many cuing differences set the stage for the child's desired and undesired eating behavior.

My first visit with the 8-month-old occurred at her house. I was greeted at the door by the housekeeper, who carried the youngster comfortably within her arms. We sat for a few minutes until the child's mother arrived from work. The youngster delighted in her mother's presence, and after warm hugs and greetings, the four of us moved to the kitchen where the child normally was given her meals. The housekeeper placed the small child into her high chair, sat in front of her, and began feeding. As Mother had predicted during an earlier phone call, the youngster ate willingly. Again as predicted, the moment Mother took over the feeding, the child's receptiveness changed dramatically. She began to squirm, cry, and push the spoon away as it approached her mouth. I quickly asked the child's mother to leave the room and requested the housekeeper to continue feeding. Within seconds, the child relaxed and quietly accepted the food. After the child ate a few more spoonfuls, I sat in the chair across from her and attempted feeding. The youngster offered no resistance. When her mother was brought back into the kitchen, the child's previously manifested squirming, crying, and food refusal commenced immediately.

As you might suspect, cues can include "items" other than food and people. They can be simple objects that have become associated with feeding. Most often, these cues set the stage for pleasurable reactions. Occasionally, however, the opposite can happen.

KIM

This experience was even more overwhelming than the following words can depict. Notice the cues that were related to eating and the child's reactions to them. I will highlight the cues for you. The child's behaviors, given the cues, will be apparent.

I sat on the floor of the child's family room and listened to her parents describe the problems they had been having for nearly a year with their 2-year-old daughter's feeding. The referral had come from the family's pediatrician, who had been aware of the child's problems and had recently become keenly concerned over the youngster's inability to maintain weight. Physical examinations had failed to uncover any reason for the child's food refusal and subsequent weight loss. The only incidents that seemed correlated with the observed changes in the child's eating habits were a slight cold and accompanying ear infection that had occurred at around the time the youngster began to show a dislike for eating. As the parents described the recent bouts with feeding, I watched the child as she played excitedly with her toys. At the moment, it was hard to imagine that the youngster could create the havoc her father had described. It didn't take long, however, to see what the parents and their daughter had lived with for many months. It began the moment I asked Mom to try feeding the child. The woman had no more than *raised from her chair* when the child's eyes abruptly changed their focus from the colorful toys on the floor to the direction her mother was walking. As soon *as the woman entered the kitchen*, the child's back arched stiffly. The youngster began to scream and thrash when *the sound of the high chair*, as it rubbed across the kitchen floor, reached her ears. Believing it would be unwise to work with the child under the present circumstances, I asked Mother to *return to her chair in the family room*. The child quieted almost instantly. With the youngster's eyes following me, I quickly walked into the kitchen, found a small spoon that I cupped out of sight in my hand, then I returned to sit near the child. Once the youngster had involved herself in play, *I brought the spoon into sight, placing it on my thigh, some 4 feet from the child*. The child's screaming began immediately. It was violent.

As was apparent, the child used the presence of the various cues to determine what and what not to do. Mother *seated in the family room* was a "safe" cue. Mother *walking into the kitchen* provided the child with an entirely different message. Again, if we can identify the relationship between cues and the behaviors that seem to accompany them, we learn something about the child, something about her perceptions, and something about what we must do to help the youngster move beyond wherever she is.

One more point before moving on to another issue involving these cues. Did you notice in the above scenario that I had been able to walk into the kitchen in plain view of the child without setting the stage for any significant reaction from her? How might you explain that? How might you define the term "neutral cue"? The concept of "neutrality" plays a critical role in a successfully developed program.

As you might expect, parents and health care workers are as much affected by cues as are the children being worked with. Later, I will begin asking you to watch carefully your own reactions to the cues the children present during your efforts at feeding. Your appraisal of your own actions and reactions will be essential in helping you develop a workable program. The following case will shed some light on the issue of cues as they affect adults involved with feeding.

BRIAN AND PARENTS

Watch the interaction between the child and his parents. Notice how they used his behaviors as cues for their own reactions. Then notice what happens when the child is introduced to a neutral cue. See if you can sense why a neutral cue, or set of neutral cues, might be an important part of a remediation program.

The near 3-year-old had been evaluated by the hospital's "failure to thrive" team because of his lack of weight gain and the staff's belief that the youngster's congenital health problems would improve with an increase in caloric consumption. Despite examinations indicating the absence of any physiological swallowing or digestive problems, the child's charted weight had not shown an increase in many months. After being requested to see the child, I phoned the parents to set up the initial meeting at my university office.

The parents arrived with Brian in hand. Almost from the moment they entered the office, the child fussed and whined despite his parents' attempts at directing him toward the toys they had brought with them. For nearly 10 minutes, I watched an interchange between child and parents that strongly suggested they were unable to exercise even minimal control over his antics. Throughout the clamor, I was informed that he was "impossible at bedtime," "impossible at bath time," and that the changing of a diaper always evolved into a frustrating, screaming wrestling match. I suggested that we meet at their house that evening.

When I arrived at the child's home, I found him sitting comfortably on a couch watching a videotaped cartoon movie. He acknowledged my presence with a full smile, then returned his attention to the movie. I stayed with him for a few minutes, engaging him in light conversation about what he was watching. I couldn't help but marvel over the differences in his present behavior compared to what I had seen earlier. The parents and I went into the kitchen and began talking. At roughly 6:00 p.m., Mother requested that the child come into the kitchen for dinner. The child's response was clear: he said, loudly and without reservation, "No!" Mother's response (to the child's verbal cue) was unexpected: she said, "Okay." When the movie ended, the child announced he wanted to watch it again.

"After dinner," Father informed, as he walked into the living room and brought the now unhappy child into the kitchen, where a plate of tuna fish, canned peaches, milk, and bread with butter awaited him. I sat quietly and observed what I suspected was a daily routine: the parents made a request as to what needed to be eaten; the child refused, most often by screaming; and the parents (when faced with those auditory cues) withdrew their requests. With each passing minute, the food on the child's plate was reduced in quantity, but not because the child ate anything but rather because one or the other parent would return to the refrigerator, little by little, what had been initially provided. Soon, the only item that remained on the plate was a single sliced peach, which the child gingerly swallowed in one gulp before returning to the now rewound movie.

"I refuse to listen to him scream," Mother informed me after we were alone.

"When he screams, you remove some or all of the food?" I asked her.

"Yes," she replied. "I can't handle his cries."

"Same at bedtime and bath time?" I questioned.

"And when it's time to change his diaper," Father interjected.

"How important is it that he eats?" I asked them both.

Casually, Mother said, "I figure he'll eat when he's hungry."

"You've been told by the doctors that Brian needs to put on weight," I responded.

"Yes, but they don't have to feed him," the woman answered, her voice reflecting her exhaustion.

"So when he protests, you react by reducing the food you expect him to eat," I said.

"That's right," she replied, as though she had no other options.

The following day, the child was brought to the hospital, where I attempted feeding him in a room equipped with a one-way mirror. Without so much as a squirm or whimper, the child, for 15 minutes, ate whatever I placed before him. When I brought his mother into the room to assist in the feeding, the child's eating stopped and his crying began in earnest. I asked the mother to once again leave the room. Although the child's crying continued for some 5 minutes, its intensity diminished once his mother was no longer present. I remained quiet and motionless, leaving the plate of food on the tray before him. When he calmed, I gently lifted a spoonful of tuna fish to his mouth. He swallowed without incident.

Later the mother asked, "What did you do?" while holding her son in her arms.

"Not much other then to tell Brian, through my actions, that I intended to respond to his cries somewhat differently than he was accustomed to. By all appearances, he didn't seem to mind my slight persistence. You see, you and your husband use your child's behaviors as cues for you to remove the food from his plate. I used the same cues to relax and keep the food on the plate before him. Again, he didn't seem to mind. In fact, I think he was sort of hungry. Perhaps he was glad to have something to eat," I said cautiously.

As is evident, the entire feeding scenario is filled with cues that influence all parties involved. It is not at all uncommon to overlook or ignore the power they contain. Shortly, I will be asking you to note if your child's eating behavior appears to differ depending upon foods, liquids, locations, or who is doing the feeding. Further, I will ask you to observe and keep track of your reactions to your child's behaviors during the feeding process. The behaviors will be cues for you, and it will be necessary to know what you do when the child cries, closes her mouth tightly, pushes the nipple, fork, or spoon away from her mouth, gags, swallows comfortably, refuses to eat what you've provided, or whatever other observable responses the youngster might manifest.

In addition to noting how you respond in the presence of your child's cues, I will also be asking you to keep track of how you respond to her behavior. That point now brings us to the issue of environmental feedback. Just as behaviors are influenced by cuing events that occur before them, so they are influenced by the type of environmental feedback the behaviors produce. Since our children are constantly being influenced by the feedback they receive for their actions, this issue, as it relates to eating, holds significance for us.

The Environment's Feedback

Recall for a moment the child who experienced searing pain whenever he ate. I named him Jesse. His eating behavior was influenced dramatically by the painful discomfort it produced: he stopped eating. Yet environmental feedback, that which was not painful but instead pleasant, eventually helped Jesse to once again eat by mouth. Environmental feedback, therefore, is an integral part of our story: when it works in our favor, as in the case where eating produces pleasant taste and/or reduction of hunger, eating is rarely a problem. Conversely, in the absence of those "natural" reactions to eating, food refusal is a near guarantee.

As we saw with Jesse, natural feedback does not always work in our favor. Painful consequences produced by swallowing or digesting must be reversed before there's any chance for "po" programs to produce consistent, successful results. Interestingly, even after natural, painful feedback has been removed, there's no guarantee eating by mouth will commence. Often, the child does not know that if he were to eat by mouth, the previously experienced discomfort would not occur. Under such conditions, a different form of feedback is required to help the child take the all important first step toward eating. It is called artificial feedback. It is what you may have to use to get the desired eating behavior started. Let's briefly compare and explain the two classes of feedback. *Natural feedback* is produced by the body; it is a direct result of the eating behavior. We are born with the ability to appreciate the sensations that come from natural feedback. No learning or experience is required to understand pain or the type of pleasure associated with eating. Artificial feedback, on the other hand, is quite different.

Unlike natural feedback that is directly tied to the child's physiological system, *artificial feedback* is provided by us. It is our words of encouragement or disapproval, our displayed emotional reactions of appreciation or displeasure, our physical reactions that may include touching, hugging, spanking, or sending the child from the dinner table, along with any number of "bells and banjos" that might be employed during feeding. The value of artificial feedback must be learned through experiences. The value is not something we understand at birth.

For simplicity, both natural and artificial feedback can be either positive, negative, or neutral. *Positive feedback* is something the child values and thus enjoys. It is something he would like to experience again. *Negative feedback*, conversely, is something the child does not enjoy; it is something the child does not wish to experience again; it is, therefore, something the child will try to avoid. Feedback that is termed neutral is essentially neither positive or negative—it is an environmental reaction that doesn't affect the child one way or another. Is this very important? Emphatically, yes. There is a very simple bottom line: *if we want a child to eat by mouth, that behavior must produce positive feedback.* The positive feedback can be artificial at first, but it must eventually be produced naturally. When eating produces negative feedback, the behavior will cease. The bottom line is, again, simple.

The Child's Perceptions of Feedback

The terms positive, negative, and neutral are, obviously, relative terms. The child determines for himself whether a particularly experienced or provided form of feedback is positive, negative, or neutral. This latter point is especially important given the fact that the feedback the child ultimately receives for his present eating efforts will have much to say about his future eating efforts. You will soon discover how crucial it is to rely on the child's judgment as to what is positive or negative for him. If you make that judgment for him, and you guess wrong, your program will not be effective.

The Child's Behavior Will Tell You of His Perceptions

You might wonder how we determine the child's judgment as to the feedback he is receiving. We must rely on the child's behavior to provide us with some notion of his perceptions. As we proceed, I will show you different ways for determining the child's perceptions. Additionally, the initial interview will provide you with several questions designed to tap the child's perceptions of what is happening regarding his eating. Every child I saw wore his view on his sleeve: he let me know immediately. With practice, you, too, will be able to figure out the child's values with no difficulty. Ultimately, if the child is not fond of eating by mouth, the task will be to show him that the behavior can produce something that he will value, something he would like repeated. You will soon discover that one of the critical components of all successful "po" programs contains an important message to the child: "Nice things happen when you eat."

Summary

1. From the moment of birth, the vast majority of children discover the joys of consuming food and liquid. For these children, the sight of a nipple or filled spoon or plate quickly becomes a learned cue that sets the stage for eating and for pleasant thoughts. Neither these children nor their parents experience the types of problems that produce serious food refusal.

2. As we have come to know, however, circumstances can occur either prenatally or anytime after birth that can disrupt a so-to-speak normal developmental eating sequence. Hospitalization, for example, can easily alter an eating routine, as can a simple cold or an uncomfortable earache. In fact, eating habits can abruptly change even though no identifiable physiological explanation can be found. Frankly, why some kids stop eating or become selective food refusers remains a mystery.

3. Since our goal is to help the food refuser discover or rediscover the joys of eating by mouth, it is essential to remember that normal eating occurs when the behavior produces pleasant tastes along with reducing the discomfort from hunger.

4. For eating by mouth to occur, the child must be an active participant in the eating process: the reduction of hunger must occur as a result of something she has done rather than what someone else has done.

5. If a child is a food refuser, each of the following must be considered as possible contributing factors:

  a. The child has no physical sensation of hunger or thirst.
  b. The child is experiencing physical discomfort when eating and/or drinking.
  c. The child is experiencing emotional discomfort as a result of previous unpleasant associations with eating or drinking.
  d. The child has learned how to adaptively manipulate her environment in order to receive something she wants—be it certain foods, or specific attention.
  e. The child has yet to learn that eating and drinking by

mouth will produce pleasant tastes and/or reduction of physical discomfort.

f. The child is confused as to what it means to eat successfully.

g. The child will eat successfully and quite comfortably for one adult but not for others.

6. For remediation of an eating problem to be successful, it is necessary to carefully note:

a. What the child is doing before, during, and after feeding. A carefully written log describing her behavior is essential.

b. How the child's environment is responding to her eating and failure to eat. Noting the type of feedback the child receives is also essential.

c. Under what conditions the child eats, as well as refuses to eat.

7. Determining where the child succeeds within the eating sequence is critical. Success, no matter how far removed from the ultimate goal of independent eating by mouth, will become the cornerstone for improvement.

8. Always consider the child's behavior in light of the environment's surrounding cues. Think in terms of how the cues are influencing what the child is doing. When looking for the key cue, be as microscopic as possible. Remember, all cues have multiple parts (food, for example, is composed of taste, color, texture, aroma, and familiarity; people have different personalities, appearances, ways of relating, and aromas). When the child behaves differently in the presence of diverse cues, try to determine which part(s) of the cues is the essential component.

9. Always consider the type of feedback the child is presently receiving for her eating efforts. The initial interview will help you obtain important historical data. While that which occurred in the past is informative, that which is happening today is vital.

10. Remember that feedback can be positive, negative, or neutral.

11. Remember, also, it is the child who decides whether the feedback she is receiving is positive, negative, or neutral. The child's behavior will tell you of her personal interpretations.

CHAPTER THREE

The Initial Interview

The questions raised and topics covered during the initial interview are basically the same for all children exhibiting some degree of feeding difficulty. While the information gathered will vary significantly, the points covered should be carefully considered regardless of the types of difficulties presently being encountered with feeding. You may need to talk with various professionals who are familiar with your child to help you obtain information specific to your particular situation. My intention is to present various factors that I have found to be worthy of investigation. When possible, I will underscore key components that will have particular importance when we move into the "exploration/acquisition" phase of the book. The points listed are intended to serve as a guide: you may find some questions or problems unnecessary given the circumstances before you.

Have Physiological Problems or Complications That Might Interfere with Eating by Mouth ("Po") Been Noted?

Our first concern speaks to the child's physical state of health as it relates to "po" feeding. You will need to determine if anything within the normal eating, swallowing, or digesting sequence is creating an organic problem and thus producing physical discomfort for the child. Usually, an evaluation by a physician and additional swallowing experts will provide information suggesting whether a "po" feeding program should be undertaken at the present time. The experts will evaluate tongue movement, palate difficulties, and hyper-gag reflexes that may affect swallowing, aspirating (fluids entering the lungs), refluxing (swallowed food traveling up the esophagus), whether food is successfully discharged from the stomach into the small intestines, and any number of other anomalies that might interfere with a normal swallowing, digesting process. While there are several medical interventions that can rectify the aforementioned and other difficulties, *our immediate concern is to assure ourselves that none of the physical problems are of sufficient severity to preclude an oral feeding program.* If there is a consensus that "po" feeding is an appropriate regimen to follow, the interview should continue. If not, the medical staff will determine what interventions will be necessary to prepare the child for a "po" program.

Prior History with Feeding

Our attention now turns to when the feeding difficulties first appeared and what events if any seemed associated with them. Some children begin to manifest problems shortly after birth; others feed well for varying lengths of time before difficulties surface. As previously indicated, unexpected hospitalizations often coincide with changes in eating; often simple alterations in routines (moving, or the presence of a different primary feeder) can have an effect; sometimes a minor cold or birth of a sibling can interfere with well-established eating. While parents rarely keep daily logs on their child's eating habits, most can pinpoint when the problems began in earnest, and can often indicate what events appeared to be functionally related.

Historical information affords a flavor of any unique circumstances that may require our attention. The professional needs to push gently the parent or caretaker being interviewed to recall any event that may have, in any fashion, played a part in the present situation. Often small details will influence what the professional may consider to be a viable approach to the child's difficulties. The purpose, then, for the gathering of history as it relates to feeding is to ascertain information that might cautiously predispose therapists toward a particular line of remediation.

What Method Is Presently Being Used to Provide the Child with Nourishment?

Now we find out whether the child is being fed augmentatively (nasal or stomach tube, etc.); whether all feedings are "po"; whether feeding incorporates a combination of the above. For "po" feeding, we need to discover if nourishment is provided solely by bottle, cup, spoon, fork, or again, a combination. When tube feedings are being employed, we need to determine how much of the total required daily intake is being provided by tube and how much by mouth. The therapist's approach will differ if all, rather than part, of the child's nourishment is provided augmentatively. The above question may help to determine whether present feeding approaches are, at best, haphazard; that the only constant is inconsistency; that the primary feeder has not been sufficiently assisted in developing a regimen that is regulated and, from the child's perspective, predictable.

Does the Child Refuse All Food, All Liquid, or Is He a Partial Refuser of Either or Both?

Of all the children I've seen, only a relative few had been total food and liquid refusers at the time I met with them. The overwhelming majority of the children consumed by mouth small amounts of either liquids, pureed solids, or table foods. The consumed quantities, however, were insufficient to maintain health and growth. (Not surprisingly, a handful of the children ate fine, so long as they were provided with what they, not so quietly, demanded.)

It is essential to determine whether the child is a partial or total food refuser. If a partial refuser, it is equally important to note carefully what the child will eat or drink, as well as how often and how much of the substances the child is willing to consume. The resulting "food menu," representing substances that provide positive cues to the child, plays a critical role in the eventually developed treatment. Little other information will provide as much direction regarding intervention as the determination that certain foods or liquids are consumed with some degree of ease and enjoyment. The preferred food menu should include all the present foods and liquids the child consumes, along with those that were consumed in the past.

Is There a Primary Feeder?

The purpose of this question is to determine how many adults are actively involved with feeding the child. While feeding is occasionally limited to primarily one adult, often several adults, either by choice or necessity, have assumed the responsibility. When considering this issue, it is necessary to note all adults, including therapists, nurses, and the like, who may be involved, no matter how infrequent the involvement may be. This determination has significance for the following question.

Is Feeding More Successful with One Adult Than Another?

As with many "behavioral" difficulties manifested by children, it is often discovered upon close inspection that the observed problems vary in both intensity and frequency depending upon which adults are present or involved.

A sizable portion of the partial food-refusal children ate considerably better depending upon who was doing the feeding. (As you recall, this observation speaks directly to the issues of cues.) The therapist should ask the parent being interviewed to recall if any adult seems to be more successful when feeding the child. If the parent is uncertain, the therapist should request that a log be kept for several days, during which time feeding is tried by different adults. Discovering that the child will eat better for one adult is great cause for optimism. Such information tells us that when certain things are right, eating is less of a problem. It will be an advantage, of course, to watch the successful adult in action. On several occasions, I have asked a child's parents to videotape each other as they have attempted feeding their child. Often the tape reveals crucial differences between the parents' approaches. At that point, an effective teaching tool becomes available.

Locations Where Feeding Attempts Take Place

Frequently, parents who are experiencing difficulty feeding their child try any number of solutions to reverse the problem. One attempt often involves changing the location of the feeding. Kitchen high chairs give way to family room couches; couches, in turn, give way to car seats placed in the middle of the house. When holding the child in arms fails to help, carrying the child while walking through the house is often tried. Some parents have given up on the family's dining room or kitchen tables and have purchased small, "personal" tables, hoping that would entice their children to eat better.

Determining where feeding is attempted and where it is more or less successful can provide additional usable information for future remediation. Location can be an important variable, particularly if the child has experienced considerable difficulty and stress with feeding at a certain location and has, thus, learned that when he is taken to that location, feeding and further discomfort are likely. Just as a spoon, bottle, plate, or fork can acquire strong unpleasant cuing properties, the location where feeding occurs can become a powerful cue, setting the stage for the child to protest vigorously even before feeding commences.

When and How Feeding Is Attempted

This issue contains three important elements. We will look at them separately:

1. The number of times feeding is attempted during a 24-hour period, and when those times occur;
2. The amount of time spent during each feeding session;
3. The overall method the primary feeder(s) employs during the feeding process.

Times per Day

It is helpful for the professional to know, both for the augmentatively and non-augmentatively fed child, the general frequency of feedings per day, along with the times during the day when those feedings occur. In the first instance, we need to know whether the child is fed three times or six times per 24-hour period, and in the second instance, it is helpful to know precisely what clock-times per day the feedings take place, be they during the child's waking day, sleeping time—as in the case of the augmentatively fed child—or a day/evening combination. Such information tells us something of what the child is used to, and what she might expect. It also tells us whether the child has ever had the chance to experience hunger or thirst.

Amount of Time Spent per Feeding Session

This element is concerned exclusively with "po" feeding time, not augmentative feeding time. While time per "po" feeding generally varies depending upon several factors, documenting the typical or average time spent feeding is important. Again, the information will tell the professional what the child is used to. If the parent is uncertain as to the typical length of the sessions, the professional should ask that the sessions be timed for a 2- or 3-day period.

Feeding Methods Employed

Unquestionably, many methods, often changing by the hour, will have been tried to reverse the child's noneating behavior, and asking someone to share what they have been doing may seem an exercise in futility. Still, the issue of methods needs to be broached in the hopes that some general techniques can be noted. Guideline questions such as the following should be explored:

1. How do you respond to the child when he puts up a fuss? Do you persist or acquiesce to the protests?
2. Is the child being forced to eat? Do you bind his arms when they are flailing at the spoon or bottle? Do you force the child's mouth open? Do you force the mouth to stay closed until a swallow occurs? Do you hold the child's head still in order to get the spoon into the mouth?
3. Have you deprived the child of food in the hopes that he will experience hunger or thirst? If so, what is the longest time period food has been withheld?
4. Do you give the child only what he agrees to eat? Do you require other foods to be consumed before the desired food is made available?
5. Is music or TV provided during feedings? Do you allow the child to play with toys during feeding?
6. Is the child allowed to eat with fingers?

7. Must the child eat unfamiliar foods?
8. How do you begin the feeding session? How do you end it?
9. Do you use any punishment or reward during feeding?
10. How do you handle the child's gagging or vomiting?
11. Are you firm, soft, patient, or tense during feeding? Are your methods any or all of the same? If so, what do you do that makes them firm, soft, patient, or tense?

Any number of other questions may be pertinent, given the historical data gathered, but one guideline is critical: the primary feeder often requires considerable assistance and support when speaking to the issue of previous and present methods. *It is essential that the professional help the parent feel comfortable sharing whatever methods have been attempted to help the child gain and maintain weight.* If the parent or caretaker senses that negative judgments will be made, important information may be withheld. Frequently, a feeding method presently being used needs to be stopped either because it is placing the child in jeopardy or because it is teaching the youngster habits that will require changing at a later date. Before any advice can be offered, however, what is presently occurring must be documented. Often, the therapist is wise to ask the parent to keep a running diary over several days, noting who is feeding, where the feeding takes place, how the child reacts to the feeding, and how the primary feeder reacts to the child's efforts. This will provide much of the needed information regarding what is being done. The diary may also provide essential clues to the following issue.

Is There an "Ideal" Situation Where Food Is Most Likely to Be Consumed with Relative Ease?

With the information gathered from the first eight items, attention can now turn to one of the most important issues to be raised during the initial interview: does an "ideal" situation exist (regarding foods, feeder, time, and location) where the child, irrespective of quantity or the foods themselves, will swallow what is placed in her mouth? You are looking for a starting point; the slightest hint from the child that tells us of the circumstances under which she feels the most comfortable and is willing to consume foods. There is no way to overestimate the value of such a finding, for it will become the building block upon which to develop a successful program. In truth, the primary feeder, because of personal involvement, may not be able to discern any such condition that sets the stage for the child's successful effort. Usually, a highly microscopic view of the eating scenario is necessary before discovering what conditions, if any, are needed to produce even a semblance of cooperative eating.

Visual, Auditory, Tactile Strengths of the Child

The focus of the interview changes somewhat as the therapist begins to note the unique characteristics of the child that might have a bearing on the type of motivational systems perhaps necessary to enhance eating. Of prime interest is to determine if the child, regardless of age, manifests a preference for visual, auditory, or tactile stimulation. Said slightly differently, does the child appear more interested in activities, toys and games that have a strong visual, auditory, or tactile component? More often than not, the child will enjoy some combination of all three, but on occasion, a definite preference can be discerned. The professional should try to determine if the child has a favorite toy; if she prefers to watch things happen, listen to things as they happen; whether sights, sounds, touches, adult recognition and affection are the most or least valued by the youngster. We are looking for objects, things, reactions the child finds to be important. The more you can identify, the greater the chances you will find something the child will both value and work hard to get. Eventually the therapist will show the child that she can get what is valued by eating.

How Much Weight Loss, If Any, Can Be Tolerated by the Child?

A few of the children I worked with were in such dire straits when I first saw them that attempting to increase hunger drive by withholding even the smallest amount of food was not medically advisable. The vast majority of the children, however, were able to lose a small amount of weight without a significant problem being created. *Prior to any intervention, the determination of "acceptable" weight loss must be made by the child's attending physician.* While it is hoped that weight loss will not occur in conjunction with any feeding program, the fact remains that minimal weight loss is a possibility. It is recommended that the child's physician be contacted to ascertain the acceptable limits of weight loss. The documented parameter, no matter how small, must be noted, and the parameter must be respected throughout treatment.

Must the Child Be Kept Off Certain Foods or Liquids?

This information is generally known prior to treatment. Nevertheless, it is wise to double check if any foods or liquids must be withheld from the child due to potential or real adverse physiological reactions.

How Does the Child Object to Eating—What Behaviors Are Manifested during Feeding Attempts That Make the Task Difficult?

I will spend an entire section discussing what I refer to as *avoidance behaviors*. These behaviors are the types of learned reactions the child manifests that make "po" feeding difficult, if not impossible. For the moment, it is very important for the primary feeder to describe in detail how the child objects to feeding: what he does that interferes with successful feeding. Does the child sway his head to avoid the spoon or bottle; close his mouth tightly; slap at the spoon, fork or bottle; scream, gag, or vomit; arch his back; struggle to get out of the high chair or away from the kitchen table; fall asleep; refuse to swallow; throw food from the tray; verbally remark that he won't eat; or behave so obstreperously that removal from the dinner table is guaranteed? Further, it is helpful to note when the avoidance behaviors begin. What cues appear that set the stage for their occurrence? Does the child begin to avoid feeding upon first seeing the bottle; upon being placed in the high chair; upon having the spoon touch his lips or food touch his tongue? It may happen that the avoidance responses may appear only (or more often) in the presence of a particular adult. It is not unusual for a child to do well for a therapist, while being much more difficult for the parent. Such divergent behaviors are critical to note. The therapist should make certain the primary feeder has plenty of opportunity to share what he or she generally sees when attempting to provide nourishment. Such information may help him or her determine how much time will be needed for purposes of generalizing one person's success to another.

Overall Compliance Issues

Although this issue may appear to have little connection with "po" feeding, it can carry considerable weight when determining intervention techniques. For many of the children I've seen, eating *per se* was not the major problem. Overall compliance to parental requests, however, was. During the initial interview, I always ask the child's parents to describe how the youngster responds to typically imposed family guidelines: does the child go to bed without protesting; take a bath or have a diaper changed without incident; stop or start an activity when verbally requested to do so? If it is discovered that a general lack of compliance is an issue, that situation most often must be remediated before a feeding program is established. Remediation targets the parents' "discipline" approaches first, after which the problems with eating can be tackled. A brief section on compliance issues (Chapter 7) offers suggestions for remediating accompanying behavioral difficulties that appear to be creating feeding and nonfeeding problems for both parent and child.

Is Now the Best Time to Begin a New Feeding Program?

Before the initial interview is concluded, it is important to determine if now is the time to begin a feeding program. Many factors need to be taken into consideration, not the least of which is the primary feeder's readiness to become immersed in a program that might be considerably different from what has occurred in the recent past. Since it is rare that a new program will reverse the eating difficulties "in a wink," the involved family members need to consider their schedules: whether guests will be visiting the home, a vacation is around the corner, the child is without fever or cold, someone is available to help with the other children or other household responsibilities, the participants' states of mind are sufficiently relaxed to endure what may (or may not) be a difficult period of time. Again the question: is it essential that feeding intervention be done now? Would tomorrow or next week be better? The question is not asked lightly. As a consultant, my job is always the easiest: I may work with the child and his parents briefly; I may visit with them several times at their house or at a hospital. But they are the ones who must participate in the program daily, often several hours during each day. They, then, must decide whether now is the time to begin or whether a few days or weeks in the future would help them become more prepared. More times than not, by the time the parents or hospital personnel contact me, they have already decided that now is the best time. Nevertheless, the option to delay briefly the onset of the program is an important choice.

Meeting with the Child

After all the above information has been noted, considered, and evaluated, and no contraindications to beginning the program have been discovered, a time is established for the professional to meet directly with the child. As simple as the aforementioned may seem, two critical decisions must precede the first meeting:

1. Where will the meeting take place; and,
2. Who will be present while the child is evaluated?

The next chapter looks at those issues, along with several others directly involved with remediation.

Summary

1. A general consensus among all parties involved needs to be reached that there exist no physiological contraindications to initiating a "po" feeding program. The child must not experience any physical discomfort from eating. If he does, a feeding program will not be successful.

2. The therapist must investigate the child's history regarding feeding to determine when the problems began, how long they have persisted, what may have been contributing variables, and any other information that you deem to be helpful.

3. Approaches will vary significantly if we learn that a child is a partial food refuser rather than a total food refuser. When a therapist learns that the child willingly eats some foods and manifests no physiological problems when doing so, invaluable information has been obtained: the therapist knows the child eats. The next step will be to determine how to increase intake, broaden diets, or generalize the successful eating behavior.

4. The therapist must determine if the child eats better for one adult than another. If it is discovered that such a circumstance exists, the therapist needs to analyze the specific approach employed by the successful adult. If possible, the professional should videotape a successful feeding session so others can learn from what is happening.

5. The therapist should get a feel for how much time is being spent on feeding. He or she needs to find out how many times a day a child is fed, and how much time (and at what times) during the day the child's physical system is without food or liquid.

6. The primary feeder should document the various approaches used to help the child eat. This helps provide a clear, precise picture of what is currently being done to provide nourishment for the youngster.

7. The therapist should determine if an "ideal" situation exists where the child will willingly eat food. If one is found, the variables involved in the ideal situation should be noted. For example:

   a. What foods are being consumed.
   b. Who is feeding.
   c. Location where feeding takes place.
   d. Time of day.
   e. Favorite toys or objects available during feeding.
   f. Overall approach the successful feeder uses.

8. The therapist should note the types of "reinforcers" or valued objects and activities the child appears drawn to. He or she should find out if the child appears more interested in visual, auditory, or tactile toys. The information will help the professional develop stronger artificial feedback programs that will be used as incentives to help the child eat.

9. The therapist must check with the child's physician to determine how much weight, if any, the child can lose during the initial phases of a new feeding program. The information will indicate how much "room" the professional has regarding withholding food in order to initiate a feeling of hunger.

10. It is very important to have the primary feeder describe, in great detail, precisely how the child behaves during feeding sessions. The therapist should pay particular attention to how the child objects to eating. What avoidance responses does the child manifest? How does he try to avoid eating? This information is essential to have at hand before beginning any program.

11. The professional must find out if now is the best time to begin a feeding program. Everyone involved must be ready. No one wants to begin a program, then end it before there's been a chance to see its overall effects.

12. Please note that before a program is begun to help a child, two critical questions must first be answered:

　　a. Where will the first evaluation take place?
　　b. Who will be present when the child is evaluated?

These questions speak to the issue of neutrality. Their importance will become evident.

CHAPTER FOUR

Exploration Phase

The exploration phase represents the first opportunity for working directly with the child. The information gathered will provide both parent and therapist with many ideas as to best help the youngster. The phase investigates many crucial points, the first of which deals with the overall goal the parents and professionals have for the child.

Overall Goal

Before a professional can make a direct evaluation of the child, he or she is best advised to take a moment to determine specifically the overall goal for the youngster. While the goal is often obvious—helping the child learn to eat by mouth—there are occasional variations:

1. Some children do eat, but not enough.
2. Others eat, but do not drink by mouth.
3. Some eat and drink, but their chosen menus are very narrow; trying something new appears out of the question.
4. Some won't allow a spoon or bottle to come within 5 feet of their mouths.

5. Others will take whatever is offered but won't swallow.
6. Some will gag or vomit immediately upon having food or liquid placed in their mouths (or placed on the table).
7. Others will wait until they've swallowed before gagging or vomiting.

Again, the goal may be apparent; still the professional should take a second to solidify precisely what he or she will be looking for and experimenting with during the exploration and subsequent phases.

The Professional's Attitude

When first seeing the child, it is important for the therapist or feeder to be calm yet forthright. To whatever degree the youngster can sense the other's emotions and state of readiness, the therapist needs to present a picture that represents preparedness and confidence. Sometimes, the above is easier said than done. I can recall the very first food-refusal child I was asked to assist: a 9-month-old who had been abandoned, literally left to die, who had already experienced numerous surgeries for intestinal difficulties and hydrocephalus (an accumulation of fluid within the cranium). The child, when discovered on the steps of a firestation, was immediately taken to a hospital, where he had remained since first being found. When I saw him, I was far from confident, further from relaxed. I remember the young medical resident looking toward me as though waiting for, and expecting, pearls of wisdom; I remember hoping that he was not able to read the jumbled thoughts that were racing (read colliding) through my mind. The physician and I were successful. Before morning ended, the child had consumed his first ever solid food: 1 ounce of baby cereal and applesauce. It was a good start.

Today, when I prepare to meet a food-refusal child for the first time, I believe that I will be able to help her. (Such is the advantage of having worked with so many youngsters.) I talk with the child, regardless of age, as though success is not problematic; rather, the uncertain variable is the time and methods it will take to reach it. So long as I am assured that no hidden, interfering, physiological problem is present, my confidence is clearly evidenced by my speech, gait, and facial expressions. Admittedly fanciful, I want the child to look at me and know that eating by mouth (if not today, then soon) is a given. After all, "Eating is fun and necessary," I say with my eyes, then quickly add, "and we're going to do it, right? Right."

The above, of course, is an attitude, a legitimate one to embrace. Nearly all the children I've seen have eventually (often quickly) improved their eating habits. Yet what I have done, methodologically, has been far from magical. That is good, for magic is difficult to replicate. Indeed, much of what I have done has been relatively simple. That, too, is good, for that which is simple is replicable. While several steps will be needed to bring about change, and sometimes a youngster's progress is two steps forward and one (or two) backwards, the prerequisite to them all is confidence. The therapist should take the first step and exude self-assurance and optimism. The child will eat—if not today, then soon.

The Parent's Attitude

I'm going to suggest that the child's parents (or the previous primary feeders) *not* be present with the child during the first phases of exploration. Ideally, the parents should be able to watch what is happening, but the child should not be aware of their presence. (If the exploration is occurring at a hospital or clinic, a room with a one-way mirror is perfect. If a one-way mirror is not available, being positioned behind a screen, or standing in an adjacent room with doors left ajar, is acceptable. If it is necessary for the initial exploration to occur at the child's home, having the parents concealed in a nearby room is also acceptable.)

Understandably, parental attitudes toward the feeding evaluation will be quite variable. Some parents will be relaxed, others very apprehensive. Some will show their emotions readily, others will be reticent to share their dispositions. Some may be flat out frightened, others nonchalant. Since it is impossible to predict with 100% accuracy how their child will react to the forthcoming exploration, it is essential that the parents be provided with an opportunity to express how they are feeling about having their child evaluated. Directly, the parents need to be asked if it is acceptable for their child to be allowed to protest or cry during the session, in the event that either occurs. If the therapist's intention is to allow the child to throw food from the tray, gag or vomit, clench teeth, flail at spoon, fork, or bottle, scream or yell, all as part of the assessment process, it is important to have the parents indicate how they will feel (and perhaps react) to such occurrences. (I have found it helpful to ask parents what I am likely to see once the child is placed in a high chair or at a table, or once an effort is made to begin feeding. Not surprisingly, the parents' predictions are usually very accurate.) The vast majority of parents I have worked with over the years have been willing to allow whatever is going to happen to occur freely. A few, however, have indicated honestly how difficult it will be for them to watch their children experience any problems during assessment. Under the latter conditions, before assessment begins, a decision must be made whether assessment should even be attempted. The professional will lose all the advantages of neutrality if he or she stops the evaluation because the child is crying, protesting, or *volitionally* gagging or vomiting.

Parental Comfort

Every effort, therefore, must be made to help the parent feel comfortable with the assessment and to allow the events to unfold naturally. Whatever the child does, she does; and whatever she does must be allowed to run its course. When the session does end, it must end on a positive note: the child, from the beginning, in the feeder's presence, must learn that any number of behaviors, other than crying, gagging, throwing food, or other forms of protesting, can bring about a cessation to the feeding process. The near-worst thing the feeder can do is to show the child that not eating will terminate efforts to feed her. If, from the parents' words and emotions, the therapist senses that he or she will not be afforded the opportunity to allow the undesired behaviors to run their course, thus preventing the professional from trying to redirect the child to more desired actions, serious consideration should be given to delaying the evaluation until a professional has had a chance to help the parents understand why the session cannot be ended on a sour note. Again, the parents must be helped to feel comfortable about what the professional is doing.

The Child's Attitude

The children's attitudes will be as variable as those of the parents. Some children I've seen have been docile and accepting, others feisty and protesting. Some, understandably, very frightened, others seemingly oblivious. Some found it very difficult to be removed from the parents, others seemed almost to relish the opportunity. Stating the obvious, we want the child to be comfortable and not frightened.

A child's sense of comfort and feeling of security may initially be quite unlikely. Make no mistaken interpretation, we are disrupting the child's routine: we are placing her in a strange place, accompanied, perhaps, by adults she may not be familiar with. If that weren't enough, we are presenting her with some familiar and possibly negative cues: a chair, eating utensils, and food, any or all of which might remind her of varying degrees of uncertainty and unpleasantries. With some exceptions, the child likely has no idea that an eating problem exists. Even if she does know that eating or its absence has created, for unknown reasons, some difficulties, it is not likely that she fully understands the ramifications of the difficulties. Having food placed in the mouth and being requested to swallow is something that happens, sometimes often. But from the child's perspective, it is just one thing, certainly not everything! There's plenty of time for other things, the child assuredly knows. "So what's the big deal?" she might ask us innocently. "What's all this furor over eating?" she might wish to pose. At the very least, she might state, "Let's get this over with so I can get on with the fun stuff life has to offer." The latter, of course, is precisely what we wish to happen. We no more want to belabor the issue than does the child.

One additional, obvious statement: all must make every effort to help the child feel as comfortable as possible. Light conversation on the part of the professional can be beneficial, as can a familiar, favorite item the youngster cherishes. If the therapist can find a new or unfamiliar toy that might spark the child's excitement, he or she might be able to momentarily, at least, redirect the child's attention from the task at hand. In truth, though, sometimes nothing the therapist will do will set the stage for the child's initial cooperation. If so, the therapist should take the lead from the child's preferences toward "getting this over with": tenderly, warmly, escort the youngster to where the evaluation will take place, and with confidence and forthrightness, get on with it.

Neutrality

I had to work with a dozen children before I appreciated fully the concept of neutrality and the enormous power established cues had on eating behavior. When I first started with the children, I almost always saw them at their homes, watching them as their parents attempted feeding in the precise location where the struggles had been occurring for months, perhaps years. There were some successes under those conditions, but the time involved seemed to stretch endlessly, as did the frustrations of both children and parents. Word of the successes soon began to reach other colleagues who also were trying to help the food-refusal children and their parents. Before long, I began to see several children within the confines of the occupational therapy department of The Children's Hospital in Denver. What struck me the most about working with the children in the new location was the shortened time it took to help the youngsters regain some interest in eating. There was less protesting from the children, and even when it did occur, its duration was brief and its severity was not as dramatic.

Neutrality's Advantages

Theoretically, neutrality (a condition or circumstance possessed of neutral cues that, from the child's perceptions, have yet to be associated with specific environmental feedback) decreases the chances that a child will be able to predict how his environment (specifically the adult feeders) will respond to the noneating behaviors. The presented cues are less familiar, thus less likely to set the stage for the food-refusing behaviors that ordinarily occur at home. Under neutral conditions, the child can't be sure what's going to happen. With feeding, this uncertainty can be a distinct advantage.

While I am not suggesting there are any absolute, hard-and-fast rules governing who must do the feeding or where the feeding must take place, my personal observations strongly suggest that whenever the opportunity for neutrality presents itself, it should be taken advantage of. The following suggestions and justifications are an attempt to convince all to seek, whenever possible, a neutral feeder and a neutral location where a feeding evaluation can initially take place.

The Feeder

Stated simply, the child's parent (or primary feeder) should not be with the child during the initial assessment/exploration process. When the child is first seen, a therapist, nurse, physician, dietitian, or psychologist should conduct the evaluation. Why? Because the child knows the parent, knows how the parent will react. Equally important, the parent knows the child, knows what the child will likely do. Together, without intent, they have developed a pattern: each reads the other's cues; each has established a way of behaving. Succinctly, the mutually known patterns and accompanying predictions must be altered. The first step toward that alteration is to have a neutral person perform the assessment. Such neutrality should be maintained until the child's eating has begun to come under the control of natural feedback (pleasant tastes and reduction of hunger) or until the professionals working with the child have devised an effective artificial feedback program that will maintain the child's efforts until the natural feedback takes over.

Question: Won't the child adjust to a newly imposed neutral situation? Won't he eventually be able to predict what's going to happen when he behaves in a certain way, thus nullifying the advantage afforded by the neutral cues?

Yes, but two issues make that inevitability unimportant. First, if the child does adjust to the new feeder and location, he will be acquiring new, more desired, eating habits throughout the adjustment process, assuming of course that the new approach is an effective one. Second, the more success the child can experience with eating, the greater the likelihood the natural outcomes of pleasant taste and reduction of hunger will begin to exercise their influence. Both issues decrease the need for further neutrality.

Location

Location for the initial assessment will depend greatly on the severity of the child's food refusal, the age and developmental language skills of the youngster, and the degree to which noncompliance and other similar undesired behaviors have come to interfere with the child's eating. Certainly if the food-refusal child is verbal, can describe the present problem and understand why remediation is necessary, the initial evaluation and subsequent treatment, barring a most unusual exception, can take place at the home. The home is also suitable for evaluation if the child's status is that of a "picky," partial food refuser rather than a "failure-to-thrive," total or nearly total food refuser. Likewise, if the major problem with the child is general noncompliance rather than only food aversion, than again the home is fine for the early evaluation. But if the child is young, with little or no expressive verbal skills along with minimal receptive language skills, with an extended history of food refusal, whose absence of weight gain or weight maintenance has placed the child's health in jeopardy, where non-compliance does not seem to be an overwhelming issue, and where the parents' efforts at feeding have failed to show any progress, then, whenever possible, the initial evaluation should not occur at the child's home. Again the issue is one of familiar cues. Everything within the usual feeding area of the home will remind the child of past experiences and set the stage for past behaviors. A hospital, department within the hospital, or clinic would be a much better location for the initial assessment. If such facilities are used, the assessment can take place with the child as an outpatient —the child goes home immediately after the evaluation—or with the child as an inpatient—the child remains in the hospital for continued assessment and treatment. The inpatient status approach occurs only under very specific conditions. If the use of the above facilities is not feasible, thus requiring evaluation at home, then a room where feeding has never taken place is a satisfactory second choice.

A large percentage of food-refusal children, again, will not require an eating evaluation in a hospital either on inpatient or outpatient status. That approach occurs predominantly with very difficult cases or when the child is already in the hospital because of severe food refusal or other physical problems. However, since food refusal can be total or near so, and thus be very serious, warranting the services of a hospital or clinic, I will spend a little more time on the issue of hospital location as it pertains to the exploration phase.

First, assume that the assessment process has occurred while the child is an inpatient at the hospital. Sometimes the feeding will take place in the child's assigned room, other times in an examination room, and sometimes within the confines of a separate department (such as occupational therapy) in the hospital. The determined location is as much a matter of convenience as anything else. As indicated, the parents will not be with the child during the evaluation. They will be close by, but not within the room. If the child begins to show immediate progress with eating, the parents may be brought into the location once the effective approach has shown itself to produce reliable, stable eating behaviors from the child. (The consumed quantity of food is not as important as the child's persistent willingness to open his mouth in the presence of the spoon, cup, or bottle, and swallow what has been provided.) The parents will practice with the established methodology while the child stays at the hospital. The practice sessions will continue until the child eats comfortably and sufficiently in the presence of the parental cues.

Second, assume that a feeding evaluation occurs within the hospital (usually within the speech or occupational therapy department), but the child is an outpatient—she is brought in from home for the evaluation, but she returns home once the evaluation has been completed. Once again, if the child begins to eat reliably during the initial evaluation, the parents will practice what has been discovered to be helpful both at the hospital and when they return home. Location at the home may not be an issue.

Third, assume that the initial evaluation has occurred at the child's home. The parents, while close by, will nevertheless be out of sight of the child. The location may or may not be in its usual place. Again, the parents will practice what the evaluator has discovered to be beneficial. A new location within the house may be tried once the child's eating behavior becomes reliable. (Reliable eating does not require consumption of large quantities of food. "Reliable" simply means that the child, willingly, repeatedly, without protesting, accepts the filled spoon, fork, or bottle. Once the child's eating becomes more consistent, once she understands the process involved in eating, the concern with quantity can be addressed.)

Fourth, assume that the initial assessment has occurred at home, and that despite the absence of the parents and perhaps the use of a "neutral" location within the home, the child's food refusing persists. Under such conditions, the parents (along with the family physician) may be requested to bring the child into the hospital as an inpatient, where neutrality, parental visits, and schedules of feeding can be more controlled. Inpatient status also allows the attending physicians and nurses to watch, more closely, the child's physiology as it relates to eating and digesting. While the latter approach may sound drastic, it can be extremely effective. Once the child is an inpatient, the assessment process is undertaken, and the parents are not present during feeding periods for several days. (They, of course, can visit with the child as much as they would like, but they are asked to leave the child approximately 30 minutes to an hour before the next feeding session begins. They can return immediately after the session has concluded.) When an effective method for helping the child has been discovered and the child demonstrates reliable eating, the parents are brought into the feeding session for purposes of practicing what has been found to work. Usually, a 4- to 6-day period on inpatient status is sufficient to gain a handle on what methods need to be employed. Once both parents and child are successful, the child is taken home, and the parents, with support, assume full responsibility for feeding.

Question: Can neutrality be achieved in places other than a hospital?

Yes. In two cases, parents were able to solicit the cooperation of neighbors who had similar-age children and who were willing to try feeding at their homes while they fed their own youngsters. The parents and neighbors stayed in contact by phone. When the "target" children began to eat more readily, their parents joined them at the neighbors so the parents could feed the children and therefore associate themselves with the successful eating. In the above instances, both neutrality and modeling of other children proved to be quite successful. I should add quickly that neither of the two target children were total food refusers, nor did they have any major physical difficulties. Rather, they were partial refusers who ate very little food both in terms of quantity and variety. During the feeding sessions that occurred at the neighbor's, the children, in addition to being fed what they were used to, were also given a very small portion of a new food that possessed a very similar cue (texture) to the more familiar food.

A State of Hunger

Regardless of location, the child should be hungry before the assessment process begins. As is obvious (and as a reminder), a child whose stomach is full is not likely to be cooperative when requested to eat more. This issue is more tricky and complex than may first appear.

A sizable number of the children I've seen were introduced to hunger by withholding the meal prior to the scheduled time for the assessment. Often, this translated into food and liquid being withheld for roughly 4 hours. Some of the children, because of constant problems with dehydration, could not afford a 4-hour period without liquids. The attending physician would order minimal amounts of liquids necessary for health to be administered during that 4-hour period, but two factors, when possible, were assured: first, the liquids would not be given within an hour of the assessment, and second, the consumed liquids would contain few, if any, calories.

For several of the children, 4 hours without food was not sufficient to produce a state of hunger. With close cooperation and approval of the attending physician (an *absolute* necessity), food was withheld for longer periods: if the child was being augmentatively fed, minimal amounts of food were delivered during the night while the child slept; and in the absence of augmentative feeding, and again with the approval of the physician, "po" feeding was withheld for 24 hours or longer.

As previously suggested, the issue and relationship of hunger and eating is not overly sophisticated. Assuming the child is experiencing no negative feedback from eating, food will be consumed when hunger sets in. Without hunger, even in the absence of any negative feedback, eating is most unlikely.

Many of the parents I worked with did, indeed, withhold food from their children in the hopes of producing a state of hunger. (Most, I must add, failed to consult with their family physician regarding their attempts. From my perspective, such is a dangerous course of action.) Despite the potentially increased state of hunger, rarely were the parents successful in altering their child's eating habits. Why? The most logical answer refers, once again, to familiar cues. The child, perhaps experiencing some slight hunger, was still being fed by his parents, and whatever associations she carried regarding the feeding scenario were basically the same, hungry or otherwise. Depriving the food-refusing child of nourishment, regardless of good intentions, should not occur unless a physician approves, and neutral feeders, preferably in a completely neutral setting, along with a carefully thought-out program, are in place.

The general rule of thumb: prior to the initial assessment, make certain the child has been without food for a time period that is both acceptable to the attending physician and likely to produce at least a minimal sensation of hunger.

Supplies

While the supplies needed during the initial assessment will vary with each child, differences often being a function of overall goals, there are certain suggestions that can cover most situations. I'll break the supplies into three categories.

Foods

For the infant, foods will generally be limited to formulas and perhaps baby cereals, the latter being dependent upon the infant's ability to assimilate the cereals safely. On more than one occasion, I experimented with thinning or thickening the baby cereals to see which consistency appeared more pleasing to the child, as well as easier for him to control once in his mouth. More often than not, a pasty consistency, one thicker than yogurt or pudding, placed directly on the child's tongue, seemed to work the best. The child swallowed the pasty cereal and then seemed quite willing to swallow a few drops of formula. (Such experimentation, of course, always occurred with a nurse and physician close at hand.) On occasion, the physicians, nurses, and I have discussed the possibility of enhancing the tastes of the foods by experimenting with added flavors that would not be contraindicated. Basically, however, the foods for the infant are quite limited.

For older youngsters who have demonstrated the ability to accept a wider range of foods, the question of variety takes on more importance. With the partial food refuser, the feeder will want to have one or two "favorite" foods available, along with one substance the child is either not fond of, or not familiar with. (Why one food the child is not fond of? Although we're jumping ahead, let me briefly explain why it is best to have a favorite and not-so-favorite side by side. We want the partial food refuser to broaden her dietary repertoire: we want her to eat different foods. To accomplish this, we want her to know that her favorite food will be available, but only after she has taken a small taste of something new. We want her to understand the same basic rule that has governed most children's eating behavior for eons: "Eat your peas and you can have your apple pie." That's Grandma's Rule. The message: "You can have what you want after you eat something else." We want her to learn a very important lesson: "You cannot have what you want unless you taste what I offer." This latter admonition must be used carefully and correctly.)

The textures of the favorite and not-so-favorite foods should be nearly the same, unless of course, increasing tolerance to different textures is a major component of the overall goal. If such is the case, the texture of the one new (nonfavorite) food should be only slightly more "granular" than the others. A child, for example, who has subsisted solely on puddings, baby fruits and vegetables, and yogurt, may find a jump to a substance with sizable lumps a difficult and aversive challenge. A consultation with a dietitian will prove helpful in determining a step between the soft and the lumpy. (I have had some success approximating the next-texture step with soft, small soup noodles, mashed potatoes that have not been creamed into liquid, Jello, or very small pieces of canned peaches as a beginning, but a formal consultation would be advised.)

For the total food refuser, the simplest, nontextured foods, such as puddings, strained baby fruits and vegetables, and the like, are the best. (For that youngster, we aren't interested in broadening his food repertoire, we're interested in getting one started.) Again, the food preference menu, obtained during the initial interview, may provide ideas (if any exist) of what the child used to enjoy. When preferences have yet to be determined, any smooth baby food will usually be acceptable during the exploration process. For the total liquid refuser, water or a juice sanctioned by the physician will do. For the partial liquid refuser, the child's favorite plus a non-favorite, also sanctioned by the physician, is necessary.

The favorite food or liquid is the most essential ingredient. Unless the child's physical state of health warrants the exclusion of certain foods (popcorn, for example, with a child who has a history of aspirating, is best avoided), the child's preference for type of food during the evaluation, should be honored. A giant step toward progress may occur quickly if the child realizes that his favorite (and familiar) food will be available to him after he has tasted what the feeder desires.

JERRY

Here's a simple example of Grandma's Rule. Notice how the child's food preference is used to help him learn the process: "You may have what you want after you taste what I want."

I saw the 11-month-old in his hospital room. Two weeks earlier, he had undergone radical, lower-intestinal surgery, and though he was recovering nicely, he had nearly stopped all "po" feeding. (During the recovery period, he had been fed augmentatively.) In the view of the surgeon and nurses, no anatomical reason existed for the sudden change in his eating behavior. The child's parents indicated that he had been a "reasonably good" eater prior to surgery; now, they added, he'll take two bites of pudding, then stop. When I asked the parents if the child had any favorite food items, even now, they responded in unison, "lollipops." They produced a paper-covered, grape-flavored lollipop: the child's eyes widened immediately. I fetched a jar of banana pudding, asked the parents to leave the room, sat down in front of the sitting child, and handed him the unwrapped lollipop, which immediately went into his mouth. After a few seconds of allowing him to lick to the candy, I took the sucker from his hand, placed a small quantity of pudding into his opened mouth and quickly handed him the lollipop. After a few additional licks, I repeated the sequence. Within moments, he handed me the sucker, opened his mouth, swallowed the provided pudding, then took the lollipop into his hand and began licking it. Once the sequence was well established, I required that he take two swallows of the pudding before receiving the candy. In less than 15 minutes, the jar of pudding had been consumed. The nearly whole lollipop was put away until the next "po" feeding.

Question: How about the older child who struggles with milk every time it is placed in front of her. Can you use the same approach? Can you say, "Have some milk, then you can have a bite of cookie?" Suppose the child says back, "I want the cookie first?"

Grandma's Rule works across all ages. Before using it, however, you have to decide how important it is for the child to drink her milk. Perhaps her diet provides her with alternative ways of obtaining the same nutrition found in milk, thus making the "power" struggle unnecessary in the first place. If you and the child's pediatrician believe milk is necessary, offering a bite of cookie for a swallow of milk is fine so long as the child likes the cookie. If the child exclaims, "Cookie first!" you can respond, "Sorry, that's not how Grandma intended for her Rule to be used." If the child protests further, you have a compliance problem. The need to resolve that issue is more crucial than the drinking of the milk.

MONA

Another example of using a favorite food to help a child try one that is different. See how I remind her of what she really wants. Sometimes it is helpful to ask the child, "Do you want . . . ?" and fill the blank in with what you know is her favorite. Additionally, notice how I "play" with the favorite bottle and the spoon, the latter being empty at first. One more thing. There's something very important that happens in the latter part of this case. Something happens with the child—specifically, with the child's understanding—that is enlightening.

When I saw the 2-year-old at her house, she was dancing around the living room holding tightly to her bottle that was filled with whole milk. In between moments where she would look at me and her mother as we talked, the child would shove the nippled bottle into her mouth, drain an ounce or so, then go about her merry way. "It's the only way I can keep her happy," Mother indicated to me as she watched her daughter. "From the moment she awakens until she falls fast asleep, she has the bottle in her hands, and, most often, in her mouth," the parent added.

"No solid foods?" I inquired.

"I try, but it is a massive struggle," Mom answered.

"Do you mind if I try something?" I asked.

"Please," the woman responded without hesitation.

The child and I went into the kitchen, where her high chair was located. (Mom stayed, as requested, in the living room.) I produced a jar of applesauce and placed it on the tray. The child immediately shook her head: the message was clear: "Forget it!"

"You're going to love applesauce," I countered lightly. "Applesauce is great," I added as I gently removed the bottle of milk from her hand. She began to cry gently. "It's okay," I said softly. "Do you want your bottle?" She looked at me and rather vigorously nodded "yes." I brought an empty spoon to her lips, allowed the spoon to graze the lips, then immediately handed her the bottle. She drank quickly as though she sensed that I was going to remove it once again. I did, but only briefly. Again an empty spoon to the lips, followed by handing the child her bottle. On the third trial, I placed a small amount of applesauce on her lips, gave her a drink from the bottle, then placed a slightly larger amount of applesauce into her mouth, which again was immediately followed by handing her the cherished bottle. Soon, the required sequence was in place: a swallow of applesauce, a swig of milk. (You get what you want after you taste what I want.) I brought Mom into the kitchen and had her watch what I was doing. Then, with Mom standing by my side, I requested that she repeat the sequence. She hesitated a drop too long with giving the child the bottle after the applesauce was swallowed. We practiced the need for immediately providing the bottle. Soon, Mom felt more comfortable with the required quick reactions. Soon, Mom sat in the chair across from her daughter and repeated the sequence. Soon, the child realized (and accepted) the established rule: the bottle would be returned only after solid foods were swallowed. A phone call a few days later conveyed that the bottle was gradually becoming less popular, and the child had begun to "supplement" her diet with more solids.

Did you catch one of the more critical components in the above example that we first covered in Chapter 2?

> the child must know what we are doing; the child must be able to predict both what we desire from him as well as what he can expect from us . . .

What happened in the above case? " . . . the child realized (and accepted) the established rule: the bottle would be returned only after solid foods were swallowed." With practice, the child was able to predict what her environment would do after she tasted the new food. The child understood the rule: "After I taste what Mom wants, I get to taste what I want." With practice, even the very young infant will come to understand the relationship between what he does and what we do. The sooner the child can predict the relationship, the sooner he will abide by its particulars.

ARNOLD

Still another example of using a favorite to assist a nonfavorite. Do you remember chocolate-drowned pancakes? Well . . . hold on to your taste buds and your personal prejudices.

The near 3-year-old would eat relatively well so long as his food was "drowned" in ketchup. As his father put it: "No ketchup, no eat!"

After a short conversation with the parents, I requested the name of the family physician. My question to her was brief: "Any problems with this child having ketchup with his meals?" Her response was equally brief: "No."

I returned to the child's parents and asked them if they had ever eaten pancakes with ketchup. "Are you kidding? Never!" they stated with turned-up faces. (The thought of such was not overly appealing to me either.)

"How about potatoes and ketchup; corn and ketchup; eggs, toast, bacon and ketchup?"

The point was becoming apparent: "We should let him eat whatever he wants with ketchup?" Mother said.

"I would," I replied. "Who knows, in a few weeks, maybe ketchup will give way to mayonnaise."

"Mayonnaise and pancakes?!!" Mom spat. "Heaven help us," she whispered.

When the child is taken to the location where the assessment process will begin, it is important to bring along every advantage imaginable. Certainly for the partial food refuser, or the child who has developed exotic tastes and esoteric combinations, go with the child's preferences. Remember, children haven't cornered the market on "rare" foods or their mixtures. Chocolate covered grasshoppers might be even more palatable drowned in ketchup.

Utensils

The utensils, of course, are quite constant: spoon, fork, bottle, cup, bib, towels, a favorite plate or bowl, high chair or appropriate-sized chair, table or similar device for the paraphernalia, and anything else that seems obvious. One additional item, depending upon the child and the overall goal, can be helpful. As I've been told, it is called a "Brecht" feeder, something I've used on several occasions without knowing its formal name. A Brecht feeder is a syringe that, in place of a needle, has a piece of tubing attached to its nippled end. The length of the hollow tube can vary, but it is usually about 1 to 2 inches long. I've used it only with young children who have a problem with liquids and who refuse to drink from either a cup or bottle. The feeder allows very small, controlled quantities of liquids to be placed in varying locations within the mouth thus enabling us to observe both what the child does with the liquids, as well as investigating whether liquid placed in certain locations enhances swallowing. The Brecht feeder, of course, is of little value if the child refuses to allow the tube to be placed in his mouth. Frequently, practicing with just a tube as it touches lips and tongue can be helpful to overcome such a problem. Due to possible aspirating, the feeder initially should be used only when a physician or nurse is close by.

Fun Stuff

In addition to reviewing with the parents the child's preferences for visual, auditory, or tactile stimulation, the youngster, when feasible, should have the opportunity of bringing into the assessment location any object that captures her fancy (size and weight taken into consideration, of course). Preferably, whatever accompanies the child should be able to fit on the feeding tray, and it should be something that both the therapist/feeder and the child can manipulate with ease. Her own favorite toy brought from home or used in the home is ideal, as is the toy, mobile, or mirror the infant or young child plays with while at the hospital.

The valued toy or object will serve a much more important purpose than mere distraction or needed support. If a favorite food or liquid is not available to help with identifying an effective method for enhancing food intake, often the toy or object will serve that purpose. On occasion, neither food nor toy will be valued by the child at the time of the assessment. While the absence of either can make the discovery of an effective method more difficult, there are, fortunately, other ways of helping the child learn to eat.

A Brief Break

Let's take a second to see where we are to this point.

1. The child has been given an absolute, unequivocal clean bill of health. No aspirating, no refluxing, no choking, no turning blue, no involuntary vomiting, "no nothing" that would contraindicate "po" feeds.
2. If circumstances warrant it, the child is in a neutral setting with a neutral feeder.
3. The overall goal has been determined.
4. Parents, unless involved in a 4 to 6 day inpatient assessment mode, are in the wings.
5. The child is comfortably, securely seated, preferably in a high chair or car seat or at the kitchen/dinner table (preferably not in someone's arms).
6. His tray and or eating table is covered with foods and/or liquids, toys or objects of interest, needed utensils, and anything believed to be advantageous.

7. The feeder is seated across from the child, preferably at or near eye level.
8. The feeder is relaxed and confident. "This is going to be a breeze," he or she says, even though the heart may be palpitating wildly.

Everyone is ready to begin. The feeder looks at the child. The feeder's eyes tell the child, "You will eat, if not today, then soon."

Evaluation of Emotional Reactions to Feeding

The next step is to determine the child's emotional reactions to the place of feeding and utensils used. From this, the therapist will catch a glimpse of any learned avoidance responses that will have to be dealt with and determine whether a procedure to help the child with his own interfering emotional reactions will be necessary. (The procedure is known as "desensitization.") Usually, this phase is extremely brief, often no more than a few minutes. Nevertheless, the therapist should go through it. Actually, if a problem relating to excessive emotional reactions is going to surface, the child won't let the therapist avoid it.

Identifying these "emotional" reactions commences the moment the exploratory feeding session begins, often with the child being brought to the location for feeding, or placed within a high chair, or being told, "It's time to eat." While realizing the limitations of an "okay" and "not okay" format for purposes of evaluating or grading a child's "emotional" behaviors, try nevertheless to "grade" the child's behavior with the "okay/not okay" arrangement. Let's say that "okay" means that the child's reactions are not severe enough to interfere with feeding. "Okay" might mean that he's sitting reasonably comfortably, somewhat quiet or only crying softly, smiling, giggling, talking, singing, or just watching what you're doing. "Not okay" might mean that he's trying hard to get out from his high chair, that his crying is loud and persistent, that he appears extremely uncomfortable and fitful, that he has begun arguing about eating, or that he has voiced a complaint of not feeling well and has begun to walk toward his room. For the moment, simply note the child's reactions and categorize them as "okay" or "not okay." If the youngster's reactions to the chair are "okay," the therapist should move to the next step. If they are "not okay," it will be necessary to go to the "desensitization" step.

Assuming the child tolerates the chair reasonably well, the therapist next checks out the child's reactions to the utensils. Here is where the therapist will likely see some strong responses. Note them carefully, particularly in terms of what they "look" like. The professional will need to check out each utensil that will be used during the evaluation session. More times than not, he or she will be looking at the child's reactions to either a spoon, fork, or bottle. Here's what to do. Take the empty spoon or filled bottle and lift it slightly from the tray or table, bringing it into the child's visual field. Note whether the child turns her head, moves her hands and arms as though pushing the utensil away, cries, closes her mouth, or demonstrates any other similar nonreceptive, avoidance reaction. Then in a series of smooth, but brief and rapid, movements, bring the utensil first to the side of the child's cheek, touching it gently, then bring it back toward the tray, then to the child's lips, touching them gently, then back to the tray, then, if possible, to the child's open mouth, touching her tongue, then back to the tray. Repeat the above sequence one more time. If the child appears comfortable with the entire sequence, this part of the exploration phase ends. However, if a nonreceptive avoidance reaction, for example, crying, head turning, or pushing spoon away, occurs with any component, note precisely what the child did. Depending upon the degree of severity, desensitization may be necessary.

Desensitization

On paper, there is nothing about a spoon or bottle (or small tube) that should evoke a strong avoidance or emotional response.

These objects (cues) at the worst should be neutral or, at best, positive. If, however, they have become associated with discomfort or fear, or if the child has learned that by manifesting avoidance behaviors a feeding session will end, the responses, discomfort, and fear become more understandable. The child, simply, is adapting to what his environment has presented to him in the past; he is attempting, as best he can, to control and functionally manipulate circumstances that he finds displeasing. Understandable, but not at all in his best interests: the child is not going to be particularly receptive to eating if a spoon or bottle sends him into a tizzy.

Desensitization is a process that helps the cues associated with feeding become at least neutral or, potentially, positive. While the process can be highly complex, it fortunately is not a difficult procedure to use when working with young children who are reacting negatively to a spoon or bottle. Implementing the process requires first that the therapist/feeder keep in mind the term *association*. The spoon or bottle has become a negative cue because of its association with unpleasant environmental consequences or feedback as they relate to feeding. Let me give you a quick example of how this association comes about. Suppose a child has been comfortably and successfully eating in a high chair for several months. The high chair, because of its associations with the successful eating, will be a positive cue. The child might smile and literally feel good when he is placed in the chair. Suppose the child develops an undetected stomach ailment: whenever he eats, he experiences pervasive nausea. Said slightly differently, whenever he is placed in the high chair to eat, he experiences the nausea. Within a relatively short period of time (varying from child to child), the sight of the high chair will create an ill feeling within the child. Through association, the once positive cue will now be perceived as negative.

The therapist's task is to change that association: he or she wants the spoon, bottle, or fork (high chair or table) to be associated with pleasant, comfortable, enjoyable consequences and reactions. During the desensitization period, I attempt to change the association by presenting, many times, the negatively perceived utensil, making certain that no unpleasant consequences occur.

"It's just a spoon," I tell the child softly, as I gently, very briefly, touch the empty spoon to his cheek or lips. "Watch as I do it to myself," I continue, bringing the spoon to my face. If a toy or stuffed animal is on the tray, I will touch the animal with the spoon while talking with the child about how much the animal enjoyed it. During all of this, I provide the child with sincere, animated, and positive verbal feedback for his efforts: "Fantastic, you let the spoon touch your cheek. That's great; you see, it's just a spoon." I might spend several minutes with this exercise, alternately bring the spoon or bottle back to the tray, then repeating the touching and verbal support. Within a short time, I will touch the child's lips once again repeating with animation, "It's just a spoon; that's great, you let the spoon touch your lips, fantastic," I might add while clapping. Then, when I sense the moment is right, most often using the child's facial expressions and body positions to guide me, I place a very small amount of pudding or strained fruit or vegetables on his lips, and as though my activity represented a common, simple, everyday occurrence, I will immediately return the spoon to the tray, tell him how well he has done, and with great effort, try to redirect his attention to a toy, animal, or some-thing he is fond of that happens to be on the tray. Most critically, the food, carried by the spoon, will touch his lips, no matter what avoidance responses he might manifest. If I have to chase his face 90 degrees, left or right, the food will end up on his lips. If I have to gently hold his face in line with the oncoming spoon (usually with a light touch of my index finger), I will do so. I will not grab or clench any part of the child's body, for under no circumstances, do I want the child to feel any more fearful than he may already be. I always figure I am quicker and smarter than the youngster: even if I have to find a small opening between flailing arms, I'll get the baby food to his lips. Further, whether he grimaces, spits out the food, rubs it off his lips with his fingers, or tries to punch me in the nose, I tell him, regardless of age or verbal receptive skills, "You did great. You ate food. That is fantastic!" I'll smile, clap my hands, do a jig, anything the child might enjoy seeing, even through his small tears. (That I am offering congratulations to the child even though he may have spit, kicked, or tried to pinch or punch, may appear confusing. A likely question might be, "Aren't you reinforcing the child for 'bad' behavior?" Initially, it is possible that spitting or other undesirable behavior might unintentionally be followed by words and actions of appreciation. Such could happen if food touches the child's lips and/or tongue at the precise time a child's thrashing occurs. The offered appreciation for the "tasting" would also occur in close proximity to the flailing. But the flailing or other equally undesired behaviors will only be significantly influenced if they consistently, or even occasionally, produce the therapist's appreciation, a most unlikely prospect. Further, after multiple repetitions, where only the "tasting" is followed by appreciation, where the flailing, pinching, screaming, or what-have-you produce no feedback from the therapist/feeder, the child will learn that it is his "tasting" that is producing the "praise," not his undesired avoidance responses.)

While employing the above procedures, I have one essential goal in mind: I want to get the youngster out of the high chair or away from the eating table for a brief period of time when he has either become more receptive to the spoon or bottle, when he has tasted the food, or both. Said slightly differently, I must find some positive action provided by the child in order to end (even momentarily) the session or trial within the session. (Swallowing the food, which would be marvelous, isn't a requirement for being removed from the chair, not at this point at least.)

Desensitization with the Infant

The youngest of infants, too, can come to perceive her feeding utensils (usually a nipple or a nippled bottle) negatively. Such negative associations can come about from at least three directions. First, if the infant has been augmentatively fed from birth, the nipple may be a foreign object. (Look at a rubber nipple closely— bring it to within a few inches of your eyes. An attractive device?) It may have no meaning or value. It may be frightening, particularly after it has been shoved into the infant's mouth quite unexpec-tedly. Second, the infant may have (or had) an undetected physical problem that flares whenever swallowing food. Since the nipple is associated with the swallowed food, the nipple may be perceived as aversive. Third, as distasteful as the possibility is, the truth is some parents have a difficult time feeding their infant. They may get frustrated quickly; they may yell; they may do worse. The association to the nipple is obvious.

Often times, a simple desensitization period, lasting for a few minutes, several times throughout the day, over several days (per-haps longer), will help the child become more receptive to the feeding utensils. For the child who has had little if any successful experience with "po" feeds, gently rubbing the gums and cheeks with a finger, first plain, then "dipped" in formula may help famil-iarize the child with "things" and food in the mouth. It may also help reduce the child's fear of the situation's newness. A wash-cloth or small towel, gently touching and massaging lips, gently placed on the child's tongue, can also facilitate the infant's state of relaxation. The infant may begin sucking on the provided finger or towel, approximating the sucking of the nipple. The entire process should be gentle and guided by infinite patience. Assume the child is either fearful of what she has already experienced, or fearful of what she hasn't experienced. Either way, check the infant's reac-tion to a finger or nipple. If the infant "backs away" or becomes frightened, the therapist should consider a brief desensitization period.

The desensitization process may take several sessions or sev-eral days, depending upon the child's history and resulting reac-tions. Its goal is to help the child feed more comfortably and be-come more accepting of the utensils that will be directly involved with feeding. The therapist will have to "feel" or "sense" when a satisfactory state of comfort or receptiveness has been achieved— the child's behavior, of course, will be the barometer the therapist will use to determine how effective the process has been. This is the "art" part of the science. The more often the desensitization process is employed, the easier it becomes to estimate its effectiveness. Sometimes, the process takes 3 minutes, then it's on to direct feeding. Sometimes, happily, the desensitization process isn't at all necessary.

The First Look at Avoidance Behaviors

A brief introduction to avoidance behaviors is necessary for four reasons:

1. The child may manifest avoidance responses during the exploration phase;
2. The avoidance responses must be dealt with effectively *the moment they first appear;*
3. From a nonphysiological, behavioral viewpoint, little else impedes the growth of acceptable eating behavior as do these avoidance responses;
4. Most important from the child's perception, the therapist can lose all the advantages of neutrality, indeed be placed in the same difficult and frustrating position as that of the child's parents, if he or she fails to act correctly, concisely, and immediately when the avoidance responses make their appearance.

Please note that I am not exaggerating the need for effectively dealing with the child's avoidance behaviors.

MARCUS

Two important points. First, notice how essential it is to "work through" avoidance responses from the moment they first appear. Second, unless there exists the most unusual of circumstances, a session, even if unplanned, must end on a positive note.

I went to the hospital to meet Marcus and his parents. Due to the child's fragile physical health, the parents had brought the youngster from their home state for consultations with several of the hospital's physicians. Additionally, they had requested advice regarding their son's persistent eating difficulties: the child, at age 7, weighed only 27 pounds. Because of the late afternoon hour and other personal obligations, my sole intention was to say hello to the family, allow the boy and me to greet one another, and set up a time for the exploration phase on the following day. The youngster, however, made my planned, brief visit impossible.

The small, pale child was sitting quietly in his hospital bed when I entered the room; his breathing was supported by oxygen delivered through nasal tubes. His parents were standing protectively close by. After shaking his father's hand, I noticed the youngster's face was suddenly filled with a lovely, boyish smile. I returned his smile, gently touched his cheek, and said hello. His offered "hi" was labored and breathy, reflecting his lifelong struggle with weakened lungs. After a few more words with his parents, I looked about the room and noticed the covered hospital food tray resting on a table at the opposite corner from where the child sat. Curious about what foods had been ordered for the youngster, I walked over to the covered tray. Without thinking or considering that what I was about to do would have any importance, I raised the tray, noticed the untouched full plate of macaroni and congealed cheese, sliced meat of unknown origin, partially covered with a thick, hardened brown gravy, and a pile of waxed, shriveled string beans, each 2 to 3 inches long. I thought to myself that the tray and its contents had been sitting, undisturbed for several hours. Innocently, and again without any intent other than to bring a little levity into the room that was heavy with silence, I lifted one of the beans with my fingers, turned toward the parents, and was about to ask them if their son had ever eaten such a thing. In all likelihood, I could have lifted a spoon or straw or napkin or anything else on the tray and produced the same totally unexpected reaction: the child, with all the strength he could muster, began to scream thinly and toss about violently on his small bed. I stood motionless, silently holding the bean in my hand. "A stupid mistake," I privately admonished myself, recognizing clearly that, by error, I was suddenly thrust upon both horns of a dilemma: if I put the bean back on the plate, the child, no doubt, would quiet and relax; if I put the bean down, I, no doubt, would lose an essential advantage I would need when working with the youngster and would be seen by the child as without determination or persistence; if I failed to return the bean to the plate, I would be obligating myself to work through the confrontation that was neither planned for nor desired by anyone present in the room. I turned to the child's mother: "I'm sorry, but unless you object, I must stay with this. If I leave without working this through, I will be taking several steps backwards."

Mother and Father looked toward one another. It was Father who spoke: "This is what he does with us; what he has been doing for as long as I can remember. Do you want us to leave the room while you do what you believe is necessary?"

I answered quickly: "No, stay where you are. I need for Marcus to see that you will not come to his rescue. I would appreciate if one of you would find his primary nurse and bring her into the room."

After the nurse walked to my side, she whispered, "All because you picked up a bean?" I nodded. Her response reflected my exact feelings: "Wow," she uttered.

Quickly, I determined the goal for the impromptu session: eating the bean was not a consideration (not a possibility in all probability); the child being relaxed and quiet in the presence of my holding the bean would do. The goal: I would leave the child and the room only after he, without crying or thrashing, allowed me to sit by his side while holding the horrid bean. I had to show him that crying in the presence of the bean would not result in my leaving. I knew it; he had to learn it.

The nurse left long before the session ended: she had more important things to do than to watch for 60 minutes as I very slowly made my way toward the child's bed, my short, forward steps occurring only when the child's crying ceased for some 15 seconds. Perhaps as much from fatigue as anything else, the child eventually remained relaxed and still as I joined him on his bed; the bean, in clear view, resting upon my thigh. "It's just a bean," I said softly to him, as I touched his wet face. "It's no big deal," I added as I stood from the bed and returned the bean to the plate. "I'll see you tomorrow," I told him with a deep breath.

The *planned* session the following day took place in his room; his parents stood in the hallway, accompanied by a social worker. Marcus began crying the moment I placed him in his high chair. The soft crying lasted nearly 90 minutes. I remained silent throughout the ordeal. When he quieted, I placed him in his bed. His parents were distraught but resolved—they had battled this many times. The next session occurred in the late afternoon of the same day. The crying lasted about 30 minutes. Marcus allowed an empty spoon to touch his lips. During the next session, held the following morning, Marcus cried for no more than 5 minutes. He ate a half jar of pudding and two bites of pancake. The following morning, he was taken to the occupational therapy department so that the session could be videotaped and his parents could watch from behind the one-way mirror. The crying resurfaced: it lasted about 20 minutes. After he quieted, he ate a small amount of applesauce and a few bites of toast with peanut butter and jelly. That afternoon, in front of the camera and the watchful eyes of his parents, he began to eat the moment I placed him in the high chair. After several bites of scrambled eggs, pancakes, and sausage, I brought his mother into the room. He continued to eat whatever his mother offered him. I left the two of them alone and stood by his father and several occupational therapists behind the one-way mirror. The child's face, as he stared at his mother, was brimming with smiles. Soon, to everyone's complete surprise, the child after swallowing, began clapping his hands as though no one in the world was more proud of him than himself. A few weeks later, I received a long-distance phone call from his mother. On the trip home, at a stop at a restaurant, Marcus had begun crying when his plate of eggs and pancakes were placed before him. Mother and Father engaged each other in conversation, not looking or attending to the youngster's behavior. Within moments, the crying stopped and the child began eating. A month later, due to his continued eating, his weight gain had become substantial.

Avoidance Behaviors

Avoidance behaviors can come in any manner or style. Since their purpose is to allow the youngster to remove himself from a situation that he perceives to be aversive or unpleasant, they can range from simple head turning to volitional vomiting. As described with Marcus, they can present themselves suddenly, at the most inopportune time. Still, as described, they must be dealt with immediately. If one or several occur during the exploration phase, they will require intervention.

Severity

Ironically, the severity of avoidance responses is not a major issue: from the child's perspective, head turning away from a spoon can be as effective an avoidance response as a full-blown tantrum. The child will manifest whichever avoidance responses have worked for him in the past.

Generalized Avoidance Behaviors

While severity is not a critical concern, the same cannot be said for the degree to which the responses have generalized. Frequently, avoidance responses will not occur with equal frequency or intensity in the presence of all feeders. As indicated earlier during the discussion of the initial interview, it is important to determine whether the child's overall eating behaviors, including avoidance responses, differ depending upon who is doing the feeding. The interviewer or therapist, as the neutral feeder, again, may not see them. If the child eats fine with the therapist, while manifesting any number of avoidance responses when being fed by his or her parents, future intervention must include a component of eliminating the avoidance behaviors in the presence of the parents. If they occur with the therapist from the moment the exploration phase begins, then intervention must first include their elimination in the therapist's presence alone prior to reducing them when the parents are directly involved.

Where the Child Succeeds: The Starting Point

Our discussion will now center on two key essentials of the exploration phase: identifying precisely where in the eating sequence the child succeeds, and experimenting with various techniques that will take the child beyond that point. For purposes of clarification, I'll set up a hypothetical eating sequence so as to facilitate our discussion of these two key components.

1. The child is sitting quietly, comfortably in the high chair or at an eating table.
2. Her head, arms, hands are relaxed; perhaps she is playing with a valued object.
3. The feeder raises the spoon, fork, bottle, or cup from the tray and approaches the child's mouth with the utensil.
4. The child opens her mouth to receive the utensil and food.
5. The child sucks, chews or swallows what has been provided.
6. Eagerly, she awaits more food.
7. At the conclusion of a determined period of time, the child has consumed the amount, as well as the type, of food the feeder had intended.
8. The youngster leaves the feeding location, engages herself in an enjoyable activity, and experiences no discomfort from feeding.

The above represents a relatively typical feeding scenario, minus a few variations a parent or therapist might include. If a child successfully maneuvered through the steps, it's hardly likely that I or any of my colleagues would be called to assist with a feeding program. No doubt the feeding behavior of the child has "broken down" somewhere along the above proposed continuum. The therapist's task is twofold: first, to identify where the behavior has broken down; second, to identify the step immediately prior to the breakdown—the step at which the child has succeeded. Let's spend a moment looking at the step at which the child succeeds.

When I work with a youngster, be she a total or partial food refuser, I always attempt to find a step within the above sequence where the child is receptive to my efforts, where she does not manifest any avoidance responses. I will work through the steps, slowly but naturally, noticing carefully the child's reactions to everything I do. If I see that a particular movement produces the beginnings of an avoidance response, I note the step that has produced the difficulty, pull back for a brief moment so I can consider which of several approaches would be best for the child. Almost always, I return to the step where the child succeeded and warmly praise the youngster for her efforts. I need for her to know that she has done well, regardless of how far she might be from the ultimate goal of eating. The fact that she sits comfortably in the high chair or at the table is a plus. The same is true if she is relaxed when food and utensils are located on the tray or table top. If she moves her head to the side when the spoon approaches her mouth, yet remains comfortable and without distress when the spoon is 6 inches from her mouth, that, too, is a plus. While it is important for the youngster to feel comfortable with a spoon held closer than 6 inches, I, at the moment, want her to know that 6 inches away is okay; it's a start, and a start is all I need.

LISA

Sometimes finding the point at which a child succeeds is difficult when working with very young children. Sitting in a high chair or allowing a spoon to touch lips may not be an issue. Pursuing the successful point, however, is just as important for the infant as for the older child. Notice the line of thinking that eventually leads to the important discovery.

The 5-month-old had been brought into the hospital for speech and occupational therapy evaluations as a result of problems associated with gagging when the youngster was provided either liquid or solid foods. Due to the frequency of the gagging episodes, the child was beginning to manifest avoidance responses (head turning, clenched mouth, and flailing hands) to all "po" feeding. During the initial interview, the child's mother indicated that the gagging was variable and unpredictable. A few days before bringing the child to the evaluation, the youngster had consumed a large jar of baby fruits, gagging only with the first few spoonfuls. The following day, however, the child's gagging, despite being offered the same food, was much more prevalent. The behavior seemed equally frequent and inconsistent regardless of food, feeder, or location. While doubting the child had an obligatory gag response, the team believed the behavior was related to some subtle variable that had yet to be discovered.

The decision was made to see if it was possible to detect what conditions were associated with a successful swallow without gagging versus a swallow that was preceded by a gag response. If such a determination could be made, the child's "po" feeding would be disrupted less often by a gag response, perhaps reducing the need for associated avoidance behaviors. The plan involved placing a few drops of food in varying locations within the child's mouth to see if any pattern existed with the gagging.

A Brecht feeder (a 12-cc syringe with a 2-inch hollow, flexible tube attached by way of a "Christmas tree"—an Addto, Inc., catheter adapter) was filled with the child's formula. With the child's head held gently, a few drops of liquid were placed on the front portion of her tongue. A gag was immediate. After a few seconds wait, drops were placed between cheek and gum, on the right side of her mouth. Again a gag was forthcoming. However, five applications of formula placed between cheek and gum on the left side of her mouth failed to elicit any gagging. That information verified that the child's gagging was not obligatory but was either related to an adjustment factor to the formula or to the location where the formula was provided. Further exploration was scheduled to see whether "adjustment" or "location" seemed more critical.

Experimenting

Once I have completed the identification of where the child's behavior is successful and where it breaks down, several options present themselves:

1. I may have to employ a desensitization process to help the child move beyond the successful step;
2. I may choose to use a shaping program with artificial reinforcement program to build upon the successful step and eventually go beyond it;
3. I may decide to ignore the step at which the behavior broke down, and begin my efforts on a subsequent step: for example, placing food directly into the child's mouth; or,
4. Depending upon the step at which the behavior breaks down and the types of avoidance behaviors the child manifests, I may choose to incorporate a combination of the above options.

Unfortunately, no magical formula exists that tells me which of the above approaches will best fit the youngster. More often than not, I am left to try one line of experimentation, see how it goes, then try another in the event the first failed to move the child beyond his point of success. (Indeed, rarely is a first idea sufficient to resolve a child's eating difficulties. Often the first will be combined with other ideas, or the first will be completely shelved in favor of something totally different. Such "multiple" experimentation did not appear confusing to the children.) During the brainstorming session, sometimes nothing comes to mind: literally, my head is a blank. Under such conditions, I will bring the child to the point where he succeeded (or wait him out until he has quieted), end the session on that positive note, remove him from the high chair or table, and review what has happened, what I have done, and consider what further options are available. The review process always begins by first noting the point at which the child was successful. I then ask myself, "What can I do to move him beyond that point?"

I must either find one small step that will bridge the gap between where the child succeeded and where the behavior "broke down," or gamble that I can bypass the point at which the child faltered and go directly to placing food in the child's mouth.

Desensitization

If the child is very agitated when first placed in the high chair, if he is crying and gasping for breath even when no utensil or food has been raised from the tray, only a few options are available:

1. I can try to calm and distract him through conversation and toys. If such redirection is going to be effective, it will occur within a few minutes.
2. I can sit quietly, positioning myself a few feet from him, and wait until the crying has ceased before removing him from the high chair. If he quiets fairly quickly and time is available, I will remove him from the chair and try to engage him in some fun activities for a minute or two, before placing him back in the high chair. I will repeat this process until being placed in the chair no longer evokes the crying. If time constraints prevent me from waiting until the child has quieted, I will remove him from the chair, realizing that redirection will not be effective, and go to the next option. (If I am "forced" to remove him from the chair, I want to make that decision as quickly as possible. When a child

cries in the chair and then is removed, he has learned a way to be removed from the chair: if I realize removing him is the "only" option, I don't want him sitting and crying for a long time before I take him out. If he cries for, let's say, 20 minutes and is then removed, he may well cry for some 40 minutes before beginning to quiet the next time the same situation occurs.)

3. I will converse with the child's parents about overall compliance issues. If it is discovered that the youngster displays similar behaviors other times and with other activities during his waking day, I will suggest that a compliance program be established along with efforts at "po" feeding. If the parents report that overall compliance is not a problem, I will ask them to review with me what they do with their child when he cries in the chair. If it is discovered that they remove the youngster from the chair when he cries, I will offer them suggestions regarding their parenting methods. Once the compliance issues have been resolved, exploration and experimentation can begin once again. If, as in the case of Marcus, the parents have come from out of state, the compliance alternative will not be available. Under such conditions, redirecting and working through the crying, as an initial course of action, may be the only option.

Shaping and Reinforcement

If the child is relaxed, or reasonably so, while sitting in the high chair, and swallowing food is not contraindicated due to gasping and excessive crying, the experimental options available to move her beyond her successful step increase significantly. Notice the four "middle" steps in the previously mentioned eating sequence:

3. The feeder raises the spoon, fork, bottle or cup from the tray and approaches the child's mouth with the utensil.

4. The child opens her mouth to receive the utensil and food.
5. The child sucks, chews, or swallows what has been provided.
6. Eagerly, she awaits more food.

If the child allows you to reach at least step 3, or to approximate it (she remains relaxed when the spoon or fork comes within 6 inches of her mouth), the "softest," most positive approach is to try shaping coupled with reinforcement. First let me explain the process, then we'll look at the specifics.

Both shaping and reinforcement are methods known to, and used by, everyone. *Shaping* is a procedure that helps an individual learn an often complex goal by teaching him the small component parts of the goal and having him experience success along the way. Teaching a child to ride a two-wheel bike, for example, is most often accomplished through the use of shaping. The child may start with a three-wheel bike, move on to a two-wheeler with training wheels, then have a parent stabilize the bike without the training wheels; and with luck and good balance, it's off to the races. In all likelihood, the child does not advance to a two-wheeler until he has mastered a bike with three wheels. Similarly, it is a rare child who hops on the two-wheeler, minus training wheels, without receiving some assistance from his parents. Shaping is a means to help the child learn more rapidly, and to better enjoy what is being taught. *Reinforcement* is feedback provided by the environment. It can be experienced "naturally," as when the riding child takes a minor spill and scrapes a knee, or artificially, when the parents shriek their joy and pride as their little one charges (maybe sways) down the sidewalk. With shaping, some children may need more time practicing one component of the complex task than other children; with feedback, some children may benefit from more reinforcement during the practice sessions than others.

When the food-refuser child shows some success at, or approximation of, step 3, I attempt to move him closer to that step or the one that follows by using both shaping and reinforcement. Suppose, again, the child shows no avoidance responses until the spoon or bottle is within an inch of his mouth. The spoon, 6 inches from his mouth, precipitates nothing in the way of avoidance. With verbal feedback that is reinforcing, I gradually move the spoon from 6 inches to 4 inches, then bring it back to the 6-inch mark. After a brief rest period, the spoon is brought to within 2 inches of his mouth. With each milestone, the child is warmly praised, and if he likes, warmly touched. As I work through these small steps, I am in no hurry, and I make certain the child experiences no sense of urgency from my movements or language. When I am successful at 2 inches, I quickly bring the spoon to the child's lips, touch them briefly, praise warmly, then return the spoon to the tray. If the child remains relaxed, having the spoon touch his lips, I will place a small amount of pudding or fruit on the spoon, and with the same movements as before, place the food on the child's lips, again praising him with warm, animated words. (Sometimes I will turn the spoon upside down so as to hide the food. This is done only when I have discovered that the child no longer manifests any avoidance responses to the empty spoon that has touched his lips, but shows some distress when he sees that food is on the tip of the spoon.)

How often I go back and forth from 6 inches to lips depends solely on the child's behavior. He will let me know if I have moved too quickly or too slowly: he will cry, fidget, turn away, or grab for the spoon. Since having food placed on the lips is a major milestone, I may, once having been successful with that move, bring the spoon back to the tray for a moment or two before repeating the exercise. Always, I will provide the child with warm feedback with each successful step he accomplishes. With a very difficult child, one who has experienced no "po" feeding for a substantial period of time, or one who appears very uncomfortable despite allowing me to place food on his lips, I may end the session immediately after I have given him the small taste of food: I remove him from the chair, bring him to the floor, and play games or simply converse. (As you will be frequently reminded, the process I am teaching him is considerably more critical than the amount of food that touches his lips.) On the other hand, if the child shows no avoidance responses when the food touches his lips, I will place food on the spoon, bring the utensil back to the 6-inch mark, then slowly but with intent, place the spoon into his mouth, dragging the food onto the tip of his tongue. Warm, exuberant praise follows immediately. I may repeat that major accomplishment once or twice more, end the session, and play with the child. Above all, I will make certain that I end the session on a positive note: the child is relaxed, and food has either been placed on his lips or tongue, if that's the step where the breakdown occurred. If the child begins to cry or manifest any other avoidance response, I will wait for the youngster to quiet, place a drop more food on lips or tongue, then immediately, with expressed excitement about his success, remove him from the high chair. If time and commitments allow, the same sequence, starting from 6 inches, will take place again in an hour or so.

The First Look at the Relationship between a Child's Behavior and the Resulting Environmental Feedback: Contingencies

Many of the children I saw did not require the above, somewhat elaborate, shaping process. Most often, an empty spoon placed in the mouth produced no serious avoidance responses. Indeed, the children, with a little insistence on my part, took food from the spoon and swallowed what was provided with no difficulty. In other words, they successfully completed steps 4 and 5 of the eating sequence:

4. The child opens her mouth to receive the utensil and food.
5. The child sucks, chews, or swallows what has been provided.

Problems become related to step 6:

6. Eagerly, she awaits more food.

When such a circumstance presents itself, I attempt to employ a "contingency," hoping to help the youngster get to a point where step 6 is a natural, comfortable part of her eating routine. Before looking at what the term "contingency" represents, a brief but important reminder is necessary. We only eat eagerly when we are hungry—when swallowing produces pleasant tastes and reduction of hunger and does not produce discomfort. This latter issue now becomes extremely critical: the use of reinforcement contingencies with a child who is either not hungry or experiencing physical distress when eating not only won't work, but will create emotional distress and discomfort for the youngster. Remember, long before step 6 becomes the sought-after goal, the question of hunger and physical pain associated with eating must be addressed.

ELLIE

Note how essential it is to review a child's history and present circumstances before employing a reinforcement contingency designed to increase the youngster's "po" feeding. Recognize from the following case how the physician decided to investigate if the breakdown between steps 5 and 6 was related to a physical rather than a nonphysical, environmental variable.

The youngster had been g-tubed around 3 months of age due to a failure to gain weight. Extensive tests failed to reveal any easily discernible explanation for the weight difficulty or the child's limited appetite. I first saw the youngster when she was nearly 8 months of age. While nearly all of her food intake was still being provided by g-tube, her parents had tried to introduce her to "po" feeds by offering fruits and puddings when they sat as a family unit during meals. The child would occasionally take a few tastes of what was offered, but the total quantity eaten by mouth would not fill a teaspoon.

I worked with the child for several weeks, noting particularly where on the eating sequence she could succeed with some ease. Although her "po" consumption had improved, the child did not appear at all pleased with what was happening: her protesting and gradually increasing avoidance responses presented themselves immediately after she consumed a few bites of pudding or baby fruit. Toward the end of the second week, the child surprised everyone by consuming her first full, 2-1/2-ounce jar of baby fruit. She ate with little fussing. Over the following several days, however, her protesting, accompanying avoidance responses, and refusal to eat returned once again. Despite the brief moment of success, the breakdown in the child's eating was clearly between steps 5 and 6. Several hypotheses were offered to account for the observations:

1. The child did not like the taste of the food.
2. The child, due to the augmentative feeding regime, was not hungry.
3. The child was experiencing some physical discomfort in conjunction with eating by mouth.

Experimenting with different tastes failed to alter the child's responses. Before manipulating the child's augmentative regime, the decision was made to reevaluate the child's physiology. A "GI" exam testing for problems with the stomach and intestines proved negative, as did a swallowing evaluation. The puzzle remained unsolved. Everything I saw pointed to some physical variable being involved, yet the tests failed to show anything remotely significant. The parents, pediatrician, speech and occupational therapists, and I met to discuss the next move. Reducing the child's augmentative feeds seemed to be the appropriate next step. Yet none of us was totally satisfied with that approach. Despite the fact that the child's swallowing was fine, that there was no aspirating, that there appeared to be no refluxing, that food drained easily from the child's stomach, there was still something about the child's behavior that said hunger was not the only issue. The pediatrician agreed. Something was inhibiting the child from moving from step 5 to step 6. Changing the augmentative feeds was put on hold. The decision was made to place the child on a 2-week regime of medication designed to ameliorate any possible discomfort from excess stomach acid. The child responded favorably almost immediately. Her avoidance responses became negligible within a few days, and the only artificial contingency that seemed necessary occurred without plan: her parents were thrilled and they showed their pleasure every time the child swallowed. The move to step 6 flowed naturally.

Back to the term "contingency." A *contingency* represents a relationship between a behavior and the environment's feedback. When a contingency is operating, the behavior always occurs first, followed immediately or shortly thereafter by the environment's feedback. When a planned contingency is used correctly, the child is expected to do as we wish before he receives what he desires. With the food-refusal child there exists one overriding contingency we want the youngster to experience and learn: when you eat, nice things happen.

Contingencies operate continuously: sometimes we have a definite plan and goal in mind when we use them (having a child take a bite of one food before he receives a bite of a different food); and sometimes they occur without intent, producing an outcome that we might not desire (a child's crying results in him being removed from the high chair). For the moment, our concern is with the intentional use of contingencies where we have a desired goal in mind.

Several important points must be considered when using contingencies to facilitate the child's eating:

1. You must identify an object, reaction, or food the child values, something he is willing to work for, something he really wishes to have or do. This will be the reinforcing feedback component of the contingency.
2. The child must be able to succeed at the required task; the behavior expected from the child must be something already within his active repertoire.

3. You must respond quickly to the child's desired behavior; when first using a contingency, the feedback component must be delivered as close to the desired behavior as possible. (This point may remind you of the shaping process. Shaping uses contingencies as part of its operation.)

Let's look at these three issues.

The Valued Object, Reaction, or Food

Determining the reinforcing feedback component is often easy: the child will let you know what she values at the moment. (As you might expect, what she values "now" may change rather suddenly.) Any toy or object she is presently playing with may suffice. Likewise, any favorite food or drink, or any specific adult reaction, such as verbal praise, clapping, or touching, may be sufficient. The therapist need only be aware of the child's value system, what is immediately exciting to her, or watch carefully what she is doing. Anything that she is doing now, assuming it is acceptable to the therapist, can serve as the reinforcement component in the contingency.

BRANDON

This case will show you why it is helpful to watch the child's behaviors carefully. The behaviors will show you the child's present values.

Some time ago, I was asked to see a 4-year-old boy who had been hospitalized due to a serious problem with his liver. One of the staff's major concerns was the child's unwillingness to eat enough food to maintain his caloric needs. The youngster seemed quite content to sit and nibble at his food for well over an hour, yet fail to consume enough of what was provided to satisfy a baby pigeon. (Out of necessity, a nasal tube was employed by the staff to provide sustenance and hydration.)

The staff had attempted to develop a "motivational/contingency" system for the youngster in the hopes of improving his eating, but their efforts had proven unsuccessful. "We can't find anything reinforcing for him," one of the nurses expressed in a voice reflecting the staff's concern and frustration. "He doesn't seem to like *anything*."

In reality, the child liked many things. The problem was that the staff hadn't looked in the right places. They failed to realize that any activity a child enjoys can serve as the contingency's reinforcement component. They had made the error of thinking that reinforcement was limited to TV, sweets, and social attention. To help them, I asked the nurse to join me at a far corner of the unit where we could watch the child without disturbing him. His activities included: playing with patients on the unit, looking at pictures from a book, carrying stuffed animals in his arms, shooting a popgun into the air, taking small sips from a can of root beer, and walking and skipping around the unit as though it was his own backyard. In less than 15 minutes, the nurse and I compiled a "reinforcement menu" that listed over 10 available choices. On the following day, a contingency system was put into effect. The child was informed that in order to have access to any of the activities on the described "menu," a certain amount of food would need to be consumed. (On the day when the system first was used, the amount of food the child needed to consume was *quite small*. We wanted him to see how the system worked before requiring the needed caloric intake. Gradually requiring greater intake of food is another example of shaping.) Once the child experienced the imposed contingencies, thereby realizing that a specified amount of food had to be eaten before he could gain access to what he valued, he began to eat more rapidly and consistently. Stable weight gain eventually allowed the nasal tube to be removed, and the child's eating soon came under the control of the natural feedback of pleasant taste and reduction of hunger.

Your first requirement when using a contingency system is,

again, the identification of what the child sees as meaningful. In truth, some children, initially, will not provide you with anything obvious that can be used as the reinforcing component. The feeding situation may be too stressful at the moment for the child to indicate what is of value. It may be that all she cares about is getting out of the high chair. If so, there's your reinforcing component.

HENRY

Note what the child values. See how it is used as part of an active contingency. Note also how the contingency is repeated so as to facilitate the child's learning of which behavior will initially be used to allow him to leave the chair.

I watched the 3-year-old for a few minutes while he sat in the waiting room of the clinic. He was calm, relaxed, and seemed to enjoy the games he and his mother and father were playing. The moment he was taken into a room where the exploration phase was to be begin, his behavior changed dramatically; as soon as he sat in the high chair, he began screaming and thrashing. Father, who had brought him into the room, tried for several minutes to calm the child, but nothing helped. I asked Father to leave the room, and I brought my chair close to the very unhappy child. The youngster's screaming persisted despite my efforts at redirecting his attention with toys, pictures, and anything I could think of. My sitting, standing, walking around and away from him was equally ineffective. My goal for the exploration phase had suddenly changed: I had to get him out of the high chair; at the moment, that was all he seemed to want. I requested one of the therapists to find the child's mother and bring her into the room. My hope was that she would be able to calm him. The contingency: I would remove him from the chair when he was quiet for 5 seconds. It took Mother nearly 10 minutes to sooth the child sufficiently to where he became quiet. He was immediately taken from the high chair. Mother held him in her arms for 30 seconds, then upon my request, placed the child back into the chair. His crying lasted about 2 minutes. Again when he was quiet, Mother took him into her arms. The process was repeated twice more: each time the child's crying lasted only briefly. On the following trial, a new contingency was attempted: After Mother placed one drop of food on Henry's lips, the youngster was to be removed quickly from the chair. The approach worked rapidly. After two successful trials with that contingency, a new one was employed: one swallow of pudding and the child was removed from the chair. The parents and I reviewed what had occurred. They were asked to practice the last contingency several times throughout the next 3-day period. Mother reported that the child began to eat better in order to be removed from the chair. Within 2 weeks, the child's eating had improved considerably: he became more willing to try different tastes. That willingness, of course, kept him in the high chair for longer periods of time.

The Child's Behavior

Since it is essential that the child learn how the contingency will work and how to experience success with it, the therapist/feeder must consider carefully which of the child's behaviors will be required before the reinforcing component is delivered. While the temptation may be great to withhold the reinforcer until after the child swallows food, such a decision may not provide success. To increase the chances the child will learn the system and gain access to the reinforcer, the therapist needs to provide the valued feedback at the child's successful starting point. This rule holds true whether the youngster has demonstrated success at step 3 (the therapist raises the spoon, fork, bottle, or cup from the tray and approaches the child's mouth with the utensil), or step 5 (the child sucks, chews, or swallows what has been provided). Notice again why it is so important to develop an eating sequence and run the child through it until her behavior breaks down. Only then can the therapist determine where the child also succeeds. If the therapist uses a contingency and the child stands virtually no chance of gaining access to what she desires, the contingency system will not only fail to work, the therapist/feeder will lose an important opportunity for gaining the child's trust.

Once the therapist and the child have practiced five or six successful relationships between her starting point and the employed feedback, the therapist can gradually begin to require more effort on the part of the child. The therapist should move slowly, again using the eating sequence as a guide for which step to tackle next. Again, the child's behavior will let the professional know whether he or she has moved too rapidly. If so, brainstorm an intermediate step between where the youngster comfortably adheres to the relationship and where the avoidance behaviors begin.

The Therapist's Response

The feeder's immediate response to the child's successful behavior is important for a few reasons. First and foremost, the therapist's quick reaction teaches the child how the system works. Most of the young children seen did not possess sufficient verbal skills to understand a lengthy explanation of how their behavior could produce the desired feedback. Active learning with the child directly involved in the process was the best teaching method available. Several successful trials where the child does something the therapist desires and receives something valued for her efforts enables her to predict more readily what consequences will occur as a result of her behavior. Second, the feeder's immediate reaction not only increases the chances the child will learn what was intended but, similarly, decreases the chances that the reinforcer will be accidentally provided for a response that was unintended. The feeder therefore needs to know which of the child's responses he or she wishes to reinforce. The feeder must attend carefully to that behavior. If the feeder goofs just a drop . . .

MARTHA AND HER MOTHER

Notice why it is so essential to be aware of which behaviors are receiving the reinforcing component of the contingency.

The child had been successfully worked with at the hospital for several days. Her "po" food consumption had increased from little more than a few ounces per day to 6 to 8 ounces per meal. After several experimental sessions, it was found that a simple contingency of allowing the child to hold a small stuffed bear after thoroughly swallowing a spoonful of food was the most effective method. Once the child's parents had practiced (with supervision) the components and subtleties of the contingency, they took their youngster home, believing, as we all did, that the child's "po" intake would, in a short time, preclude the need for further augmentative feeding. As always, I asked the parents to call me after several feedings at home so I could be kept abreast of the progress. As sometimes happens, I didn't hear from them for nearly a week. When the phone call finally came, Mother informed me that the child's progress had slipped substantially. She indicated further that her husband had been called out of town ever since they had arrived home from the hospital, and she believed that the father's absence had been responsible for the child's setback. I visited the child's home the following day. I asked Mom to do a feeding session so I could watch what was happening. My thinking was that while the child may have been upset at her father's continued absence, Mother had likely, inadvertently, changed something within the contingency system. The "slight" error became evident quickly. The child remained comfortable and relaxed when placed in the high chair. She appeared to anticipate the filled spoon as it was brought to her mouth. The first swallow occurred without incident. Mom brought the spoon back to the jar, filled it once again with food, *then* handed the child the stuffed animal. (The child was sitting quietly when given the bear. Technically, sitting quietly was being reinforced.) The filled spoon was placed in the child's mouth, and as the youngster swallowed what had been provided, Mom took the animal from the child's hand and placed it on the tray. (The desired behavior, swallowing, had occurred. Unfortunately, it resulted in the animal being removed.) The child displayed her displeasure at having the animal removed and began to cry. Quickly, Mom handed her the valued bear. (The child was crying when she received the bear. Technically, crying was being reinforced.) As the next spoonful was being swallowed, Mom once again removed the animal. When the crying started, the animal was handed to the child. In short, the contingency system had been changed—not so subtly. I asked Mom to stand behind me as I remodeled the correct delivery method. Immediately after the child swallowed, she was handed the animal. After a few seconds of "playtime," the animal was placed on the tray, the spoon of food was placed in the child's mouth, and as soon as the swallow occurred, the animal was once again handed to the child. Once the correct flow was reestablished, the child ate willingly and comfortably. No further crying was observed.

Again, *if the feeder isn't careful when attending to the delivery of the reinforcer, it is easy to accidentally begin to teach the child to do the opposite of what was intended.* Providing a stuffed bear when a child cries, then removing it when the child swallows, will not help the professional achieve his or her goal. Until the child's eating behavior comes under the influence of natural feedback (pleasant tastes and reduction of hunger), artificial systems will be necessary. When using artificial systems, the therapist/feeder must constantly be aware of which of the child's behaviors are receiving the desired feedback.

Testing the Limits

Inevitably, at some point during the exploration phase, the therapist will want to "ask" the child to do more than he might desire. Said slightly differently, the therapist will want to take the child beyond his successful starting point in order to see if some insistence on his or her part will facilitate the child's "po" feeding.

In a sense, the professional will be testing the strength of the child's acquired avoidance responses in order to see if the youngster is willing to relinquish them. This "testing the limits" must be done with care, for the child will be pushed beyond his present comfort zone. Several issues need to be considered. Let's look at these issues, as well as some justifications for this experimental component.

    1. Neutrality.
    2. Introducing positive contingencies.
    3. Methods.
    4. Returning to the successful starting point.

Neutrality

It is mandatory that "testing the limits" be attempted by a neutral feeder in a neutral location. Chances are great that the original primary feeder, either by intent or accident, has tried previously to push the child beyond the successful point in the eating sequence. Chances are equally great that the effort hasn't worked, that indeed all that has been accomplished is a further strengthening of the child's avoidance responses. A neutral feeder in a neutral location may not set the stage for these avoidance behaviors: the child may be more inclined to try something new in the presence of such neutral conditions.

Introducing Positive Contingencies

The purpose for testing the limits is twofold: first, it is a way to show the child that positive feedback will be forthcoming when he behaves in a prescribed fashion; second, it represents the therapist/feeder's initial attempt to "break through" the acquired avoidance responses.

As said earlier, many of the children seen had not experienced

positive feedback for gradually moving through an eating sequence. Most often, the children's primary feeders jumped several
of the steps, concentrating their efforts at placing food in the
youngsters' mouths regardless of the children's successful starting
points. Frequently, the results were less than desired: the children
learned new ways to avoid feeding entirely; the parents became
more frustrated; and neither party experienced any enjoyment
from the eating experience. From the parents' perspectives, feeding time was destined to become a battle even before it started.
From the children's views, the only "positive" component was that
eventually the battle would end.

While far from guaranteed, testing the limits can provide the
child with an opportunity to experience something he values, as
well as showing the youngster how to access that experience. The
hope is that once the child learns that something positive exists
and learns further what he must do to receive that which is valued,
the child will be inclined to jump several of the steps in the eating
sequence.

Methods

The therapist should have available for immediate delivery a
valued object, toy, or desired food or drink. If the therapist is going
to feed with his or her right hand, the valued object is best kept
either in the left hand or on the tray. *Immediate delivery is essential.*
Fill a spoon with pudding-type food, and place the food into the
child's mouth. If necessary, gently prevent the child's head from
moving away from the spoon as it approaches the mouth. Also if
necessary, use enough pressure to place the spoon into the child's
mouth in the event the youngster attempts to keep her mouth
closed. During this test, the food must enter the child's mouth. The
moment, and for emphasis let me repeat, the very moment the
food is in the child's mouth, the therapist/feeder must present the
child with the valued reinforcer. The professional should then sit
back and warmly praise the youngster: "You're eating, that's

great!" If the child likes clapping, singing, and dancing, do any or all. The child must know that something spectacular has been accomplished. After a few seconds of rest, repeat the above.

The professional needs to watch the child's reactions very carefully. He or she is looking for the slightest degree of receptiveness: the child quiets a bit; her swallow is easier; her movements to avoid the spoon decrease a bit; her facial expressions are less tense or fearful; she makes a move toward the valued object; or any similar responses that tell the therapist the child is willing to continue. If the therapist does sense that the child is prepared to stay with the procedure, the child must not be overloaded: a spoonful or two of food, then rest; another one or two, then rest again. The time period for the testing session should be brief. The therapist wants the child to experience the relationship between swallowing and receiving the valued reinforcer, then the therapist wants the youngster out of the chair and onto activities more appealing. After a half hour or so, the above procedures can be repeated, but the repetition period should also be brief, successful, and as enjoyable as possible.

Returning to the Successful Starting Point

As can happen, the testing-the-limits phase can prove to be ineffectual. Due mostly to the strength of the child's avoidance responses, the process may not move the youngster any closer to the goal of consistent "po" feeding. If the therapist concludes that the testing experiment will not be of benefit, he or she will need to bring the session to a quick end. At the same time, the professional will need to end it on a positive note: by allowing the avoidance behaviors to terminate the session, the therapist will be making them more resistant to future interventions. If possible, return to the child's successful starting point and end the session when she manifests the behaviors associated with that level. If such is not possible, simply remove the child from the high chair, irrespective of what she is doing, thus ending the session. At that point, it will be helpful to reevaluate the employed contingencies to see if a stronger reinforcement component can be identified, consider overall compliance as an issue, as well as review the child's present state of hunger.

Conclusions

The eating problems manifested by nearly all of the children I've seen over the years were rarely, if ever, due to one factor or etiological (causative) variable. More often than not, a combination of factors brought the children to their present eating conditions. All of the total food-refusal children had some physiological complication that served as a precursor. Compliance issues, some minimal, others severe, quickly entered the picture while the physical problems were being treated. Invariably, the combination of the two conditions produced resistance to, or avoidance of, "po" feeds.

One of the purposes for the exploration phase is to determine, when possible, which factors—physiological, compliance, or feeding—appear to stand in the way of persistent, appropriate "po" feeding. While all three factors are nearly always involved in some manner or kind, the following are some soft guidelines to help with discriminating if one factor appears more crucial, at the moment, than the others.

Physiological Problems

By the time the children were brought to my attention, the vast majority of their physiological difficulties, if such ever existed, had been diagnosed and remediated to whatever degree possible. There were times, however, when attending physicians were unable to rule out conclusively the existence of additional physical difficulties that might have been playing a role in a child's food-refusal behaviors. While far from exacting, the exploration phase's data and observations provided the justification for further medical tests. On several occasions, further medical tests revealed problems that required remediation before a nonphysiological, "behavioral" approach was begun. The following are some issues to consider when the existence of physiological factors remains problematic.

1. If a child's eating is acceptable in the presence of one adult but not another, or in the presence of one location but not another, the problem is rarely physiological.
2. If the child eats one food acceptably, but avoids others of similar consistency, texture, taste, and ingredients, the problem is rarely physiological.
3. If the child readily takes one or two bites of food,

   a. and then stops abruptly despite not having eaten or consumed liquids for 6 to 12 hours (plus or minus a few),
   b. or fusses and whines excessively, perhaps arching his back,
   c. and the patterns have occurred for several days,
   d. and the youngster manifests no overall compliance problems,
   e. and the primary feeders have not altered their approach significantly,

   then further medical investigations are likely warranted. (Two of the seen children had "reflux" problems that had gone undetected during an initial evaluation.)

4. If the child eats acceptably, then vomits while relaxing after the meal, medical tests should be considered. On the other hand,

   a. if the child gags or vomits as food is brought to his mouth,

  b. if the gagging and vomiting occurs in the presence of one adult or location and not another,

  c. if the parent consistently ends the meal as soon as the child vomits, and that pattern has occurred for a substantial amount of time,

then environmental/behavioral problems are likely involved.

5. If the young child consumes 40 ccs of food and does well (30 ccs equals 1 ounce), but vomits after eating 60 ccs, and that pattern has been persistent, and compliance problems are not an issue, and the vomiting occurs despite the feeder and location, the problem is most likely physiological, and, as with the above suspicious physiological signs, needs to be evaluated by a gastroenterologist.

6. If the child is being fed augmentatively, eats fine for a while, then stops abruptly, and compliance, personnel, and location are not seen as problems, medical tests are again likely warranted. (One child had problems with gas building up in his stomach that he was unable to expel; another had difficulty with undetected aspirating.)

7. As we know, eating "should" occur if:

  a. the child is hungry;
  b. he is experiencing pleasant tastes from his food;
  c. no known physical pain or stress is associated with eating;
  d. the reduction of discomfort from hunger is satisfied by "po" feeding;
  e. compliance and cooperation are not an issue.

If the above five factors appear to be operating in our favor and the child continues to avoid feeding, the child's physiological system must be reevaluated. While no guarantee exists that something physiologically significant will be discovered, the search is essential. Over a dozen of the children seen were found to have a

reflux or swallowing problem after their initial physiological evaluation had proved negative. Physiology can change. It pays to
have it checked and rechecked. However, if either a, b, d, or e are
suspect, then our etiological investigations must turn to something
besides physiological variables.

General Compliance Problems

Compliance problems that interfered with eating were most
likely to be found with children 18 months of age and older. Almost without exception, these children (as old as 8 years) were
healthy with no present physical condition that appeared to be
involved with the eating difficulties. During the exploration phase
(which, because of the children's behaviors, often lasted only a few
minutes), these children would protest from either the moment
they were placed in the chair or the moment the spoon or fork was
raised from the tray or table. Their vociferous protests were un-
affected by verbal redirection, ignoring, or shaping. No available
reinforcer was powerful enough to establish even the most minimal of contingencies. Their crying, screaming, or verbal complaining began almost before the evaluation began. Several of the older
children starting gagging as soon as they saw their food. From
their parents' accounts, bedtime, bath time, diaper change, putting
toys away, following simple directions, along with any number of
other "daily" behaviors evolved into power struggles that left the
parent exhausted, and the child further from such family concepts
as cooperation and responsibility. Most often, these children
would eat enough to maintain body weight, although their diets
were limited generally to the fewest of foods, some having little
nutritional value. Frequently, these children's parents had little to
say about when or where food would be eaten, or what or how
much would be eaten.

When these children's eating behaviors were evaluated in the
hospital or clinic, it became apparent early on in the exploration
phase that little would be accomplished. When the initial evaluation occurred at the children's home, the same problems of non-

compliance and vigorous protesting were observed. It was apparent that before a "po" feeding program could be investigated, the children's parents would need to change how they responded to their youngsters across all settings involving everyday living. With the parents' approval, a behavior management program was established to offer assistance in dealing with the compliance issues. Often several weeks of home intervention was necessary before the children realized the importance (and value) of their cooperation. Once the parents learned how to influence their youngsters' behaviors more effectively, the children's eating difficulties were reevaluated.

General Feeding Problems

By far, the major portion of problems associated with food refusal with the children roughly 18 months of age or younger had little to do with compliance or present physiological complications. Minor problems with compliance and major difficulties with health were likely earlier factors that had been mostly resolved by the time the children were evaluated during the exploration phase. The children, when placed in the high chair, were generally calm and relaxed. Their protests, usually involving crying, head turning, and pushing the spoon or bottle away, were minimal and brief. Many would allow a spoon to enter their mouths; some would even swallow a few spoonfuls without difficulty. What "fears" existed were easily resolved through a few moments of desensitization. Problems that appeared more directly involved with food refusal related to:

1. The absence of hunger (due to continuous augmentative feeding);
2. Not realizing that eating by mouth would reduce the feeling of hunger (due, again, to experiences with augmentative feeding);
3. Experiencing neither "natural" nor positive "artificial" feedback as a result of "po" eating;

4. Memories of unpleasant associations with eating and parental reactions or painful physiological feedback;
5. Inconsistent feeding regimes;
6. An abundance of moderate (although sometimes intransigent) avoidance behaviors that impeded change and growth;
7. On a rare occasion or two, a parent's willingness to allow the child to eat the same food (singular!) every meal, everyday;
8. A few minor compliance issues that were reversible with a simple contingency;
9. A few minor parental problems involving their misuse of contingencies;
10. A few minor parental problems involving inconsistency;
11. A few minor parental problems involving expecting a little too much, a little too soon (frustration, no doubt, the culprit).

Fortunately, the problems associated with the above general feeding problems are relatively easy to resolve. At the same time, problems that are accompanied by physiological difficulties can also be resolved once the physical issues have been remediated. Likewise, problems that are compounded by compliance issues can be successfully influenced once the compliance issues have been addressed.

The Next Step

What needs to be done once the exploration phase has ended depends largely on what has been discovered. Many issues that often seem unrelated to disturbed physiology need attention. As such, we will spend the remainder of our time checking and rechecking avoidance, compliance, and other issues that are likely unrelated to a physiological base. The first item deals with the oft-mentioned avoidance behaviors. Assuming there are no physiological factors interfering with "po" feeds, and assuming that a state of hunger can be guaranteed, avoidance behaviors represent one of the more major hurdles parents and professionals will have to overcome. Once they have been resolved, the child's "po" feeding problems may vanish.

Summary

1. The therapist should have a well-established goal in mind before beginning the exploration phase. Discuss with all parties involved whether eating, drinking, quantity of either, generalization, or whatever, are to occupy the professional's present efforts.

2. It is essential that the child's behavior be allowed to run its course during the exploration phase. Parents should know why it is necessary to allow whatever is going to occur to occur naturally and unimpeded. If the child's protesting is allowed to terminate the session, the advantage of neutrality will be forfeited. The child's crying (most often an avoidance response) will be reinforced.

3. Neutrality offers a means to decrease the chances the child will use familiar cues to predict what will happen given his eating behaviors. In a sense, it offers the best opportunity of starting "fresh": new faces and places. The "newness" can be a powerful ally.

4. The child's parent, therefore, should not be present during the initial assessment/exploration process.

5. The therapist should use simple, easily consumed foods during the exploration process. Avoid foods that, due to consistency, will stay within the mouth for a long time. With the partial food refuser, have at least one non-preferred food along with one or two favorites. The therapist should use the favorite food as a "reinforcer" for the nonfavorite.

6. Have available any objects in which the child shows interest.

These items, toys, games, or the like will also be used as "reinforcers." Allow the child to bring to the session something of value, something that he would like to hold tightly.

7. If the child shows any degree of "emotional" discomfort toward a feeding utensil that the therapist believes will interfere with feeding, a brief desensitization period should be considered, where the utensil (empty in the case of a spoon or fork) is brought to the child's mouth several times without being associated with anything unpleasant. With very light, pleasant words, the feeder should tell the child, regardless of receptive skills, that "this" is just a spoon or bottle; that there's nothing to worry about.

8. If it is necessary to desensitize the child to any particular part of the eating process, make certain the component being targeted is associated with pleasant moments.

9. As soon as the child appears the slightest bit receptive or quiet, place a small amount of food substance either on the child's lips or tongue. This move to the mouth is critical: the feeder must make sure the food touches the child's lips or tongue; the feeder must avoid stopping his or her efforts because of the child's protest. The child must know that his head turning or arm thrashing will not prevent the food from reaching his lips. Once the food makes its contact, let the child know, exuberantly, that he is eating.

10. Keep in mind that children (and infants) who have had very limited or no experience with "po" feeds have all the right in the world to be leery of spoons, bottles, bibs, and the rest of the paraphernalia. A gradual introduction to the articles and foods should be considered.

11. Be especially alert to any avoidance response that the child displays. Note it for future reference, but deal with it the moment it appears.

12. During the initial explorations with the child's eating, the therapist should pay particular attention to where on the eating sequence the child succeeds. Identify clearly the successful starting point.

13. Eventually, the therapist must find either one small step that will bridge the gap between where the child succeeded and where the behavior broke down, or gamble that it is okay to bypass the point at which the child faltered and go directly to placing food in the child's mouth. A good deal of the remaining time with the child will be devoted to finding the best method to help the child jump the hurdle that is presently impeding his progress. The therapist may try to desensitize the child to what is bothering him; he or she may try to use reinforcing contingencies where the child can have access to what he desires after he tries what the therapist has in mind for him; or if the therapist feels that the child's behavior will not be redirectable at the present time, he or she may end the session (on some semblance of a good note) and discuss, with the parents, a compliance program.

14. When using a contingency system, it is essential that the therapist/feeder have at his or her disposal something the child truly values at the moment. The therapist will provide the valued object or reaction once the child has successfully completed whatever has been determined to be his starting point. Such an approach guarantees that a child will experience success with eating and, more critically, begin to learn the major contingency you're attempting to teach him: nice things happen when you eat.

15. Before attempting to move the child beyond his starting point, make certain the exercise is run by a neutral person in a neutral location. The therapist does not want the child to be able to predict what will happen when he fusses or, perhaps, takes a swallow of food. Any successful movement beyond the successful starting point must result in a powerful payoff for the child: he must know that he has accomplished something spectacular.

16. Every food-refuser's noneating behavior must initially be assumed to have an organic base. An error in that direction can only cost a little time and money. Initiating a "po" feeding program when a physical problem relating to eating exists will create further problems for both the child and his primary feeders. The child who experiences pain from eating will find an avoidance response that will enable him to avoid the discomfort. That is a given. The longer the avoidance response needs to be used, the stronger it grows.

17. The most common nonphysiological problems relating to food refusal are:

   a. The absence of hunger (due to continuous augmentative feeding);
   b. Not realizing that eating by mouth will reduce the feeling of hunger (due, again, to experiences with augmentative feeding);
   c. Experiencing neither "natural" nor positive "artificial" feedback as a result of "po" eating;
   d. Memories of unpleasant associations with eating and parental reactions or painful physiological feedback;
   e. Inconsistent feeding regimes;
   f. An abundance of moderate (although sometimes intransigent) avoidance behaviors that impede change and growth;
   g. On a rare occasion or two, a parent's willingness to allow the child to eat the same food (singular!) every meal, everyday;
   h. A few minor compliance issues that usually are reversible with a simple contingency;
   i. A few minor parental problems involving their misuse of contingencies;
   j. A few minor parental problems involving inconsistency;
   k. A few minor parental problems involving expecting a little too much, a little too soon (frustration, no doubt, the culprit).

   With parental cooperation, the above are resolvable in a relatively short period of time.

CHAPTER FIVE

Avoidance Behaviors

It is the avoidance responses of the food-refusing children that we now must deal with. No other nonphysiological variable has as much impact on the child's noneating behaviors as her acquired avoidance responses. If we can help the child work through the acquired avoidance behaviors, we will get her to eat, more often than not.

It is helpful to realize that children have not cornered the market on these types of responses. Behaviors that are termed *avoidance responses* are an integral part of living. Without them, our lives would not only be shorter, but more uncomfortable than necessary. Understanding the function of avoidance responses will help us replace those that are interfering with a child's eating. We can see avoidance responses in operation on any given day:

1. Before jumping into the shower or bath, we test the water to make sure it isn't too hot or cold. Taking the second or two to touch the water with our fingers is an example of an avoidance response. Such actions enable us to avoid being unexpectedly scalded or "frozen" by the water. More often than not, we test the water because on a previous morning we've stepped into the shower without testing and have experienced an unpleasant sensation.

2. When making breakfast, we (and our children) stay a safe

distance away from the fire or heating element. Keeping our hands, arms, and faces away from the heat source is an example of an avoidance response: we do not wish ourselves or our youngsters to be burned by the element or splattering grease. We've likely experienced the latter once before and wish to avoid having the same experience again.

3. When we drive to work and notice the roads are wet or icy, we are more cautious about braking and accelerating. We might even drive within the posted speed limit. Our careful driving is a further example of avoidance behavior. The memory of a previously experienced "180-degree" spin or a fender bender sets the stage for our greater alertness and slower driving speed. The sudden skid or accident is not something we wish to have repeated.

Adaptive, Learned Behaviors

Avoidance behaviors are adaptive responses that have been learned through experience. More often than not, they have been acquired after we have been burned or battered by hot water, hot pizza, a "hot" boss, an ice-covered step, or an expensive speeding ticket. Likewise, children acquire avoidance responses after they, too, have experienced an unpleasant reaction to their behavior. Try as we might to teach our youngsters the dangers that life occasionally presents, the children may have to learn themselves that working stoves can be painful and that trees in the way of a moving bike can produce scrapes and bruises.

The Development of Avoidance Behaviors

Since environmental feedback that is perceived as aversive is, by definition, something best not experienced again, all of us will do what is necessary to avoid such a repetition. We may find a response that enables us to avoid undesired environmental feedback by experimenting with various options, or we may be taught by friend or parent how best to avoid what we'd rather not experience. While any two of us facing the same unpleasant scenario may acquire different ways of dealing with it, whatever actions are chosen will have a common base: they will occur because we have learned that our actions allow us to avoid what we have interpreted to be unpleasant or frightening. If our chosen action even momentarily helps us avoid what we wish not to experience, chances are good that we will repeat that action or behavior when the same (or similar) situation presents itself in the future. Indeed, the following principle underlies the acquisition of all avoidance behaviors:

> If a child discovers that one of his behaviors enables him to avoid what he'd rather not experience, whatever he did that enabled him to avoid the experience will begin to occur more often when he is once again faced with the same situation. (Specifically, if a child discovers or learns that headturning, thrashing, arguing, or volitional vomiting enables him to avoid eating, the learned behavior will occur more often when he finds himself being asked to eat.)

While the above "axiom" may appear relatively straightforward, two prominent inclusions must be recognized: first, not everyone sees the same circumstances as being equally aversive or, in fact, aversive at all; second, particular acquired avoidance responses may not, in the long run, be beneficial to the individual.

Perceived Aversiveness

Nothing appears to be universally unpleasant to everyone: that which is seen as aversive by one person may be valued and sought after with great zeal by another. One individual (adult or child) may do whatever is necessary to have an experience repeated, while another may do whatever is necessary to avoid the same circumstances. (One child may clamor to get into a high chair, while another may clamor to get away from it.)

How can we discover if a situation is viewed by a child as

unpleasant? Short of asking the individual to list her likes and dislikes, the only way for us to know whether a situation is or is not perceived as aversive is to watch the individual's actions: if the individual appears to be working hard to avoid experiencing an activity, there is likely an element of aversiveness within those circumstances. Given our topic, a child will not work to avoid a high chair or work to avoid eating unless an element of aversiveness or unpleasantness is presently perceived by her. Equally important, a child will not continue to display her avoidance responses unless she has discovered or has been taught that those actions will enable her to avoid the aversive scenario. Said slightly differently, if the child discovers that her responses *work*, they will continue to occur.

Undesired Avoidance Responses

Not all of our acquired avoidance behaviors are seen by others as being equally admirable or desirable. We rarely hold in high respect people who lie or cheat, yet lying and cheating are avoidance responses, and both often enable the perpetrators to avoid something they wish not to experience. Avoidance behaviors, therefore, can be judged either desirable or undesirable by others. While such classifications are easy to invoke, it is equally easy to forget that such behaviors, despite their sometimes unseemly character, are adaptive (they have been learned through experience or have been taught unwittingly) and purposeful (they enable the individual to avoid something he perceives as aversive). While such "justifications" may not make the responses more palatable, they may help to make them more understandable.

Avoidance Behaviors with Food Refusal

Avoidance behaviors with food refusal can also be either desired or undesired. For example, we want our child to tell us when his stomach is full, that if he takes one more bite of food he will "burst." Such a verbal disclosure is a form of avoidance behavior: we want our child to have a response available that will enable him to avoid becoming ill as a result of eating too much. Over time, we may have taught our child other desirable avoidance behaviors (besides turning "green") that let us know when eating is no longer desired. Putting a fork down by a dinner plate, sitting back in a dining room chair, gently pushing the plate a half inch or so away, grimacing slightly, softly closing the mouth as if to indicate that nothing else will be allowed to enter, all impart the same message: "I've had enough to eat!"

Less desirable (from an "outsider's" perspective) is the response, "I'm full," when such is not the case. So also is pushing the plate away (abruptly), throwing a fork (or food) to the floor, clamping lips shut when food is offered, screaming rather than sighing, grimacing not so unnoticeably, arguing, pouting, crying, or doing all (and more) nearly simultaneously. Yet desirable or otherwise, acceptable or otherwise, the responses, like their more palatable "cousins," are adaptive and full with purpose: something "out there" is aversive, and the youngster, for the moment, wants no part of it.

The Acquisition of Avoidance Responses

Common avoidance responses manifested by food-refusal children are most often acquired slowly, without notice. They start out as small protests, hardly seen, hardly of concern. Sometimes they remain barely noticeable, producing little if any interference with eating. Frequently, they dissipate for lack of need or purpose: that which initially was perceived as aversive (a new food, for example) becomes no longer bothersome (after trying it the child finds it enjoyable). Other times, however, due to circumstances that go unnoticed or unresolved, they begin to gather strength and character that significantly interfere with a typical eating regime. These latter responses eventually become the focal point of a therapist's intervention. Picture the following condensed scenarios.

COLEEN

A child with no physiological problems. Notice the following behaviors of the child: releasing nipple, no longer sucking, head turning, and crying. Most critically, notice the effects these behaviors have on the child's mother and what she does when the child manifests the above responses. Ask yourself, "What cues provided by the child does Mom use to stop her efforts at feeding or to end a feeding session?"

An infant has been consuming food from bottle or breast. Her stomach is full, and she pulls her mouth from the nipple. Mother offers the nipple once again, but the baby does not suck. Taking the cue from the child's behaviors, Mother ends the feeding session. The same sequence of events occur over many days. The child learns that releasing the nipple and not sucking terminates feeding. Both responses are developmental avoidance behaviors: they are the means by which the child tells her mother that she does not wish to eat anymore. Sometime later, solid foods are introduced to the child. The child finds the baby fruits enjoyable, but she doesn't like the cereal. When Mother places the fruits in her mouth, she swallows; when she begins to place the cereal in her mouth, she turns her head away. Mom tries the cereal for several meals. Each time, the child turns her head from the spoon. For the time being, Mom feeds her child liquid formula from the bottle and baby fruits. She does not try to feed her cereal. The child's head turning is an avoidance response. She is learning that to avoid cereal, she needs to turn away from the spoon. A few days pass. Mother decides to once again try the cereal. More determined, she chooses not to accept the head turning: she will hold her daughter's head gently and place the cereal in her mouth. The child turns from the cereal but to no avail. She cries slightly. After swallowing the cereal, the child is given a spoonful of fruit. She readily accepts it. As the cereal approaches her mouth, she turns her head once again, feels her mother's hand on her cheek and begins to cry. Mother places the spoonful of cereal on the tray and offers the child her bottle, which she accepts willingly. Once more cereal is tried. The child does not turn her head. Instead, she begins to cry before the spoon reaches her lips. The spoon returns to the tray and fruit is provided. Crying is a new avoidance response. The child begins to learn that head turning no longer works; crying, however, does. After consulting with the pediatrician, the cereal box is put away and Mom introduces a suitable replacement the child enjoys. The head turning and crying cease. The brief skirmish with the avoidance behaviors ends. Both Mother and child are satisfied.

BETSY

A postsurgical, augmentatively fed child. Again, notice which of the child's behaviors end feeding efforts. Note how one behavior leads to another; that when one behavior loses its effectiveness, the child will find one to take its place.

For the first 10 months of life, the youngster eats fine: her growth and body weight increase within acceptable limits. Prior to her first birthday, the child requires hospitalization and surgery. During a 1-week recovery period, the child experiences only augmentative feedings. At the end of the week, "po" feeding is instituted along with the augmentative feeds. When the bottle's nipple is placed in her mouth, she chews on it for a moment then begins to cry. The nipple is removed. The child learns that crying results in the bottle being removed. A spoon with solids is tried. The child's crying terminates that effort. The avoidance response of crying becomes stronger. A new feeder decides to ignore the crying: the filled spoon is placed near the mouth; the child closes her lips tightly. The spoon is retracted. The feeder decides to force the spoon past the child's closed lips. The child pushes the spoon from her mouth with her tongue. The spoon is placed on the tray. The feeder persists: the tongue is held down by the spoon and the food is placed on the tongue. The child gags as she swallows air and food. The spoon is put away; "po" feeding stops, and the child receives all her nourishment from the augmentative feeds. The growing "chain" of avoidance responses is:

a. Crying
b. Closed lips
c. Tongue thrust
d. Gagging.

(Remember, the one that works will occur more frequently.)

MATHEW

Undetected physical discomfort from eating. Note how the environment's reaction to the avoidance behavior is responsible for the response's continuation. Notice what happens to the "final" avoidance response after the physical problem has been resolved and the child is brought home.

At some point during development, the child has begun to experience pain when eating. Prior to that time, the child was a good eater. Now, every swallow produces discomfort. The child quickly learns that the sight of the high chair, food, spoon, bib, or bottle signals feeding; the child has learned that feeding means pain. He cries at first. At first it successfully enables him to avoid "po" feeds. Head turning works also, for a while, as does thrashing and screaming. Each enables him, momentarily, to avoid being fed. The "po" feedings, however, persist. While sitting in the high chair, he gags when food is placed on his tongue. That, too, works for a while. Then he vomits while in the chair. That terminates feeding. Soon he begins to vomit before being placed in the chair. The problem producing the discomfort is identified and remediated. The child is returned home. He continues to vomit prior to being placed in the high chair. The avoidance behavior is well established.

RYAN

An older, "picky" eater with no physical problems. Notice how the development of avoidance responses remains relatively constant regardless of age, experience, and verbal skills.

The 5-year-old does not like the spaghetti his mother has prepared for his lunch. He complains of its appearance and smell; he says he doesn't like to eat worms. Mother, taken aback, removes the pasta and offers the child a cheese sandwich which is readily eaten. The child learns that complaining about food results in its removal. At dinner, he doesn't wish to eat what is provided. He voices his disapproval of the meatloaf, indicating that he wants a cheese sandwich. His father reacts quickly: "You don't have to eat the meatloaf, but you will get nothing else. You will also not watch television tonight," the father adds. The child learns that in the presence of his father, complaining does not result in the removal of food. The child sits quietly, deciding what to do. Tears well in his eyes. Father notices the tears. "Okay," Father says, "you can have a cheese sandwich." The child learns that tears bring him what he desires. Later in the week, the child cries after being informed that he will have to finish most of his dinner before being dismissed from the table. His parents inform him that his tears "will not work."

Upset, the child yells, "I always have to do what you want."

Father excuses him from the table, pointing out, "You cannot sit here and scream." The child learns that screaming enables him to avoid finishing his dinner. The child is learning the value of avoidance responses. He will continue to use them as long as they work.

As the above cases depict, a predictable sequence underlies the development of avoidance responses relating to "po" feeding:

Step 1. Quite innocently, the child may not be hungry, he may not like the food that is offered, he may be feeling a little ill, or he may be experiencing some discomfort when swallowing or digesting his food.

Step 2. When the spoon, fork, cup, or plate is provided, the child purposely uses whatever cognitive and/or motor resources he has in his repertoire to indicate that he doesn't wish to eat. He may randomly experiment with various behaviors, or he may use a desirable response his parents have previously taught him. By pure chance or accident, a new response, not previously a part of the child's repertoire, may occur—the child may gag or vomit because too much food has been placed in his mouth, because the texture of the food is different from what he has been used to, or because of nausea, nasal congestion, or the like. By chance, he may use his tongue to push the bottle or spoon from his mouth; he may whimper; he may turn his head; he may push food from his tray; he may clamp his mouth shut; he may scream, argue, or offer justifications for why he shouldn't have to eat what was provided—any or all by accident.

Step 3. Having seen or heard the child's response, the feeder stops feeding or no longer requires the child to eat, perhaps briefly, perhaps completely. With or without intent, the feeder, by stopping the feed, has shown the child that his response will bring an end to the eating sequence.

Step 4. Depending upon the child's health, state of hunger, or food preferences, the youngster may signal that he wants more food, different food, or that he's pleased the feeding has stopped. If the latter is preferred, the child will begin to learn what he must do to avoid further feeding. Depending upon how quickly the child learns and how often (and consistently) the feeder's actions are repeated, the youngster's avoidance behaviors will become more established and more likely to occur in the future when he no longer wishes to eat.

Types of Avoidance Responses

I suspect I have seen every possible avoidance response related to food refusal. If one remains that has not been manifested by the children I've worked with, I'm not sure I want to see it. I've watched the smallest tongue serve as a barrier against an equal size nipple; I've seen tiny lips quiver as they strained to prevent nipple or spoon from entering a mouth hardly larger than the nipple itself. I now spend considerable time thinking about which shirt or pants to wear before seeing a youngster for an evaluation. I've observed youngsters work terribly hard to gag or vomit; I've watched them plan where and with whom they choose to throw up—I've been the recipient more times than I care to count. I've listened to screaming and yelling, the volume of which would compete with a turned-on rock band. Many of the children displayed considerable skills with hand–eye coordination: batting a utensil away from a suddenly closed mouth occurred with the skill of a major league ball player. I've learned how much food a youngster can "squirrel" away in the side of his mouth; how strong his jaw muscles can be; how persistent persistence truly is. Of all the avoidance responses seen, the one that will always stand out as being the most unusual (and one of the most difficult to work with) was the "open-mouthed child." This child, when walking around or playing with toys, kept his mouth closed and swallowed, without difficulty, his own saliva. But if you placed one drop of liquid or food in his mouth, a drop no larger than the head of a pin, his mouth would not only open, it would stay open. I watched him walk around and play, with mouth open, for over an hour. It would remain open until he was convinced the one drop had slithered down the side of his face. Satisfied, he would close his mouth, swallow his own saliva, and go about his merry way.

Avoidance Responses Serve a Purpose

Regardless of the type of avoidance responses acquired through trial and error or teaching, they all served an important purpose for the child. Redirecting or eliminating them required that their purpose be identified. The purposes for these responses probably are limited to the following familiar items:

1. The child does not wish to eat because he isn't hungry.
2. The child does not wish to eat because eating causes him physical discomfort.
3. The child does not wish to eat because of "emotional" associations with previously experienced feeding methods.
4. The child will not eat because he has learned that noneating, rather than the opposite, produces desired attention from his primary feeder.
5. The child will not eat because he doesn't like what's being offered.

Let's quickly review these issues.

1. The child with a full stomach or a feeling of fullness has no need to eat. The insistence upon further feeding will likely be perceived as aversive. The cues associated with the feeding (primary feeder, location, utensils, etc.) will acquire aversive properties. Such circumstances are particularly frequent when augmentative feeds are necessary and employed throughout the day and evening. The purpose for the child's food refusal: avoid stomach fullness that has reached a point of being uncomfortable.
2. The child who refuses to eat when pain is a direct result of eating is simply manifesting adaptive avoidance behaviors. The circumstances that are producing the pain need to be remediated before "po" feeds are attempted. Requiring a child to eat when eating produces pain will, again, only solidify avoidance responses. Purpose for food refusal: avoid physiological pain.

3. If the methods employed to feed the child at an earlier time were unpleasant or uncomfortable, the child may well believe that future methods will also be aversive. Desensitization along with new, more comfortable methods are necessary. Purpose for food refusal: avoid repetition of fear-producing eating methods.

4. & 5. Occasionally, a child has learned that he can control or influence family dynamics through feeding. Under such circumstances, the issue of feeding becomes less of a concern than the family's methods of relating to the child. The parents, hopefully, will benefit from assistance directed at helping them learn new ways of dealing with the child. The purpose for food refusal: enables child to receive parental attention otherwise not provided, or enables the child to eat what he alone desires.

The Child's Avoidance Responses Are Telling You Something

Since avoidance responses are adaptive, learned behaviors, they have the power to tell us that something within the child's environment is not supporting "po" feeding. Avoidance responses alert us then to the fact that further investigation of the physiological and social environment is necessary.

"D"

The following child was beset by many problems; her case was most difficult and frustrating. It is being presented to remind us all that if an initial physical exam has failed to show any reason for the absence of feeding, this does not automatically mean that a physical problem is not involved. In the face of a persistent eating problem, occasional exams are often essential. Further, notice how stubborn avoidance responses can keep us on our toes: they are telling us something.

I met with the 7-year-old's parents and listened as they described the physical problems their daughter had experienced. She
had developed normally until the age of 4, when a malignant brain
tumor was discovered. Shortly after successful surgery and recovery, a second brain malignancy was found. In conjunction with
surgery and chemotherapy, the child lost the use of her lower
limbs. During the multiple medical interventions, the child had
been fed augmentatively through either a nasal tube or Broviac
tube (the latter a line directly into the child's venous system
through which nutrition and fluids are provided). Prior to the surgeries, the child had eaten acceptably, although she never had an
enormous appetite. The child's primary physician had suggested
that a try at "po" feeds was in order. He had been unable to find
any physical reason why the youngster shouldn't be eating by
mouth. I met with the youngster at her home. As though she had
been aware of it for months, she told me that if she could recover
her appetite, she wouldn't need the tubes any longer; that if she
would eat, she would feel better; that if she refused to eat, she
could become sick. When I asked her if she knew why I was meeting with her, she looked toward me with her large, deep brown
eyes and said, with an innocence reflective of her age, "You're
going to help me get my appetite back." It was as though she had
no doubts about my ability to do so.

From the initial interview, taken with parents and child present, it was learned that two major problems seemed to occur when
the child tried to eat by mouth: she would complain of nausea, and
she would occasionally vomit. Neither response occurred every
day; both seemed unattached to any clearly discernible environmental cues. In addition, the complaints of nausea and the occurrences of vomiting rarely, if ever, occurred when the child realized
that in order for her to participate in a family outing, the food
placed on her plate would need to be consumed. The observations
seemed to point toward an obvious conclusion: the child was using
the verbal complaints of nausea and her occasional vomiting as a
means to avoid eating. (Of the many things these children have
taught me over the past years, one lesson has been invaluable: be
cautious of what appears so obvious.)

For 2 weeks, the child was provided with the opportunity to earn any number of valued activities and objects by simply eating the food her mother provided. On some days she would eat (and earn the "reinforcers"); on some days there would be no eating (and no reinforcement). On the noneating days, complaints of nausea and bouts with vomiting were prevalent. Something obviously wasn't right. Avoidance behaviors serve a purpose, and these actions just didn't fit. The decision was made to reevaluate the child's gastrointestinal system once again. The results of this investigation were different from earlier examinations. The physician discovered that food, once entering the child's stomach, would remain within the stomach's walls for much longer periods than expected. The physician suggested that the child's nausea and vomiting were understandable. The physical problems took precedence over continued "po" feeds.

"E"

While avoidance behaviors often signal the presence of a physiological problem, the behaviors may also tell us that something within the child's external environment may need investigating. The purpose for an avoidance response may relate to the relationship between the child and his parents.

The 3-year-old's history was unusual: the child began vomiting before he was 1 month old. Mother sought no assistance for the behavior for several months. When finally seen by a physician, the child was dehydrated and undernourished. Once hospitalized, the child was provided with fluids and calories sufficient to return him to a relatively healthy state. Despite multiple interventions from many professionals, the vomiting persisted. At age 3, and once again hospitalized due to malnutrition and dehydration, the child would vomit some four to six times per day. Physical examinations failed to disclose any present reasons for the behavior.

Despite a great deal of offered support by the hospital's staff,

Mother seemed hesitant to share much about the relationship she had with her child. She thought she had somehow "given in" to the child over the years when he vomited, but when pushed to provide some examples, she said she was unable to do so. Since the avoidance behavior was present, it was serving some purpose. The staff decided to look at the child's social, interactive environment to see if some external variable was involved with the vomiting.

For 3 days, the staff took turns watching the child and mother interact with one another. Careful notes were taken to document any consistent pattern that might have existed between the child's vomiting and the antecedent cues and following consequences. While preliminary analysis of the collected information showed that some of the vomiting seemed unattached to any specific cues, a sizable portion of the behaviors occurred immediately after a request made by the child was not immediately granted by the mother. The data revealed, however, that the child was quite likely to receive what he requested after he had vomited. In addition to further medical tests, a plan was drawn to help the child's mother understand the impact she was having upon her child's behavior.

A good rule of thumb is to view the existence of avoidance behaviors as red flags. They do not occur capriciously. They have a purpose. In general, they tell us that something associated with feeding has gone awry. Specifically, they alert us to reevaluate the child's physical and environmental systems. Avoidance behaviors are adaptive. They have been either taught directly by a malfunctioning physiology, or taught unintentionally by an unknowing environment. In either instance, the source of the behaviors must receive attention.

EDWARD

Frequently, parents are not aware of the behaviors they are teaching their child.

The 4-year-old's weight had fallen below the 15th percentile, and the child's pediatrician and Mother were both becoming concerned. Mother insisted that the child was experiencing some physical problem that was responsible for the absence of weight gain. "He eats well," she repeatedly told the pediatrician. "Something is wrong," she would state unequivocally, "and you're not finding it." Despite multiple examinations, no physical reason could be discovered to account for the child's weight problems. I met with the single mother to see if I could help. The initial interview disclosed that the youngster's noncompliance behaviors had become so pervasive that he would do what he wanted, when he wanted, throughout the day. His mother no longer was able to exercise any control over his behavior. As of late, the noncompliance had spread to eating. He was eating foods that contained very few calories and even less nutrition. Any limits set by Mother would be met with a barrage of avoidance responses, most in the form of screaming and tantrums. The mother would quickly give in to the child's protests. After meeting with her twice, I asked her to keep a log of her son's behaviors, along with her reactions to what he did. Once she read her own account of the daily interactions between herself and her child, she understood the degree to which she was influencing his behaviors. That recognition led to major changes both in terms of her approach and her son's behavior.

Eliminating Avoidance Responses

Several of the children I worked with relinquished their acquired avoidance responses once the aversive conditions were removed. For those children, intervention required little more than changing their augmentative feeding schedules so as to increase hunger and/or medically remediating physiological conditions that were producing pain and discomfort in conjunction with swallowing and digesting. The "natural" feedback from pleasant tastes and

reduction of hunger were the only experiences the children needed
to once again begin persistent and appropriate "po" feeding.

The vast majority of the children, however, required more
intervention than the above. Their avoidance behaviors (and emotional reactions) had become sufficiently established to necessitate
varying degrees of behavioral remediation. In addition to assuring
a state of hunger, several sessions were initiated to work through
the manifested avoidance responses.

Working Through Avoidance Behaviors

In order to work through the avoidance responses, it is necessary for the therapist to set the stage for them to occur. By doing
so, it becomes possible to show the child that the responses not
only are no longer necessary, but will no longer work. Having
them occur, of course, will likely require nothing more than placing the child in the feeding position.

An important reminder. The phrase "no longer necessary" assumes
that we have done everything possible to assure that all aversiveness associated with eating, swallowing, digesting, has
been resolved. The child, thus, is hungry; no pain or discomfort will come about as a result of eating; and the feeding
methods will be without prolonged, undue distress. The
phrase "no longer work[s]" means that the child's avoidance
responses will no longer bring the entire eating session, or a
singular eating trial—where spoon or bottle is brought to the
child's mouth—to an end. Effectively working through the
avoidance responses is significantly enhanced if general compliance issues have been resolved or at least reduced to a point
where the child can be more readily redirected or relaxed. This
latter concern will be looked at in a moment.

When the therapist works through avoidance responses, he or
she actually goes right through them. It's as if they aren't occurring. Let me bring back the previously listed eating sequence.

1. The child is sitting quietly, comfortably, in the high chair.
2. His head, arms, hands, are relaxed; perhaps he is playing with a valued object.
3. The therapist raises the spoon, fork, bottle, or cup from the tray and approaches the child's mouth with the utensil.
4. The child opens his mouth to receive the utensil and food.
5. The child sucks, chews, and/or swallows what has been provided.
6. Eagerly, he awaits more food.
7. At the conclusion of a determined period of time, the child has consumed the amount, as well as the type, of food the feeder had intended.
8. The youngster leaves the feeding location, engages himself in an enjoyable activity, and experiences no discomfort from feeding.

Assume that the child's avoidance responses do not begin until a filled spoon approaches his mouth (step 3). When "going through" the responses, the following happens. The child can turn his head, cry, or attempt with his hands to move the spoon or bottle away, but the therapist quickly places the filled spoon into the child's mouth. The moment the food enters the child's mouth, the feeder provides positive feedback immediately. The child can gag, offer verbal complaints, or volitionally vomit, and the therapist treats those behaviors as if they did not occur. If the child vomits, he or she is cleaned quickly, and the therapist continues with the sequence. The professional does not allow the avoidance response to delay for even a second the spoon from entering the mouth. Again, the therapist goes right through it as though it had never occurred. Suppose instead, the avoidance responses begin earlier, when the child is placed in the high chair (steps 1 or 2). The therapist's attitude is the same: if the child cries or thrashes about slightly, they are treated as if neither happened. The therapist has two options. First, he or she can work through the fussing in the high chair by ignoring it. Second, quite matter-of-factly, he or she can place food on a spoon and place the spoon into the child's mouth. Let's say the child swallows a first bite, but manifests the avoidance responses when the second spoonful is offered (step 6). The therapist's stance, attitude, and accompanying verbal statements are straightforward: "I'm sorry, but you must have a second bite." When the second bite (and swallow) occurs, the therapist provides some form of positive feedback: "Thanks!" "Great job!" or, "Now you can have a sip of milk."

Time Must Not Become an Issue

When working through the avoidance responses, the therapist must make sure that time does not constrain his or her efforts. There is no guarantee that a child will do what the therapist wishes within a 30-minute period. During the working-through phase, the therapist needs to have as much time as will be required to produce a positive response from the child, rather than an avoidance response. If time is a problem, "working through" can make matters worse. Note the following scenario. For purposes of neutrality, a therapist has chosen to become the primary feeder. (This may occur either in a hospital setting, where the child is an inpatient or outpatient, or at the child's home.) As usually happens, the therapist has a sizable case load. She has a maximum of 45 minutes to spend with the child before having to see another. All the prerequisites are in place: the child is hungry, the therapist is assured the child will experience no physical pain from eating, favorite foods and toys are available, and the session will be carried out in a neutral location. The therapist has speculated that the child's present avoidance responses are habituated behaviors that began months earlier when the youngster legitimately experienced negative associations with "po" eating. Now, since the "cause" for the discomfort has been rectified, the responses are vestiges from past experiences; they are no longer necessary. The child, however, does not know that "po" eating is safe and will be enjoyable. The therapist believes if the child will take a shot at "po" feeds, he will find it to be a comfortable, highly pleasant experience. The therapist readies herself . . . as does the child. The filled spoon is brought to the child's mouth. Without hesitating, the child begins to throw a tantrum. The therapist knows that if she backs off due to the child's screaming, the screaming (already an avoidance response) will be strengthened. Determined, the therapist places the food into the child's mouth, praises the youngster exuberantly, and calmly brings the spoon back to the tray. The child swallows and quiets. As soon as the filled spoon is once again raised, the child's crying begins again. The therapist, rather than repeating her earlier actions, holds the spoon an inch or so from the child's mouth, waiting for the child to take the spoon into his mouth. Instead, crying , sometimes soft, sometimes forceful, continues. The minutes pass quickly (although the opposite may be perceived). The therapist notices the present time and remembers that she has another child to see. She places the spoon on the tray and removes the child from the high chair. The session has ended. Results: since the child's crying occurred in conjunction with the session's termination, the likelihood is very strong the child will cry again (perhaps for twice the present length of time) the next time "po" feeding is attempted. Because the crying has been reinforced (from the child's perspective it was the one action that caused the session to end), the avoidance response will become more resistant to change.

If the avoidance response has been identified as crying or tantrums rather than head turning, gagging, swatting, or volitional vomiting, it is essential to have available enough time either to allow the crying to completely run its course or to manufacture a positive response that can be used as the basis to end the session. If the child's present avoidance behavior terminates the session, the behavior will become more persistent.

Number of Exposures

It is near impossible to predict how many exposures or trials of "going through" the avoidance behavior will be needed before the responses begin to weaken. Some of the seen children gave up their avoidance responses almost immediately: once they experienced the absence of discomfort from swallowing, experienced the full sensation of pleasant taste, and experienced the joy from the available artificial reinforcement that was provided after they swallowed, the avoidance responses disappeared after no more than two or three "forced" exposures. They learned that eating could be fun, that their protective avoidance responses were no longer necessary. Most of the children, however, required repeated trials that incorporated carefully used contingencies and shaping throughout many small meals, over 2 or 3 days, before they began to relinquish the responses. Some of the children gave up their avoidance responses rather quickly, only to manifest them again at some later point in time. When those children were seen, almost always at their homes, it was discovered that some variable within the planned sequence of remediation had been altered inadvertently. The variable was either an incorrectly used contingency, a breakdown in consistency on the part of the parents, a sudden loss of hunger on the part of the child (due to illness or alteration of augmentative feeds), or an incorrectly developed process due to an error or oversight made during the exploration phase. More times than not, once the variable was identified and altered, the child once again relinquished the avoidance responses.

Ending the Feeding Session on a Positive Note

When working through avoidance responses, it is essential that a session or trial end on a positive note. Just as it was with the "exploration" session, the child must learn, as quickly and with as much consistency as possible, that her avoidance responses will not bring an eating session to an end. Frequently, the therapist will need to manufacture the required positive action: if he or she can see that the child will not swallow another bite, then food placed on the tongue, the child becoming quiet or handing you the spoon, or any other "approximation" of swallowing may have to suffice. By noting the child's avoidance behaviors, and remembering at what point of the eating sequence the child has been successful, the therapist will be able to determine an acceptable, alternative response if one is needed. Ideally, however, the professional will want the youngster to repeat whatever part of the goal behavior she has been working on before the session ends. (Note: a positive response used to end a session can be any action the therapist perceives to be desirable and one that will promote, rather than interfere with, future efforts at "po" feeding. As indicated above, being quiet for a moment may be all that is momentarily possible. If that's not possible, the therapist could have the child hand her a bottle or spoon or fork. The therapist could have the child touch the bottle or plate—anything that the therapist requests that the child complies with is enough. The essential element is that the therapist controls which behavior will bring a session to a close.)

Showing the Child the Avoidance Behaviors Are No Longer Necessary and Will No Longer Work

The therapist will have an easier time of working through and "going through" the avoidance responses by keeping in mind the essential purpose of this phase: he or she wants to show the youngster that her avoidance behaviors are no longer necessary (because no physiological aversive factors exist), and that they will no longer work (they won't be allowed to end the feeding session). Further, by working through the responses, the therapist, actively, will be able to show the child that her cooperative, desired behaviors will produce an event, action, or object that she values.

Providing Alternatively More Desirable Behaviors

For the child to learn that her avoidance responses aren't necessary, that they won't be accepted, and that there are ways for her to gain access to what she values, she will need to have at her disposal a clear understanding of what it is that she is expected to do. The therapist/feeder cannot "pull" from the child the only responses (her avoidance behaviors) that have worked for her in the past without providing alternatively more desirable behaviors. *The child must know of some desirable means to gain access to the artificial reinforcers the feeder will be using.* As she experiences the process that shows her how to gain access to that which is artificial, something interesting happens concomitantly: she begins to test the waters involving "po" feeding. By doing so, she gives the "natural" reinforcers a chance to take over.

The Acquisition and Maintenance Phases

We are now ready to put most of what we have looked at into some logical flow. As we discuss the acquisition and maintenance phases, I will be able to share the many subtleties that have shown themselves to be important components of the process that can enhance successful "po" feeding. As indicated many times, the parent or therapist must converse with the child's primary physician before undertaking any part of what I will discuss. The physician can then suggest whether it is medically prudent to try any or all of what will be presented.

Summary

1. Avoidance responses represent one of the more crucial variables interfering with "po" feeding. Helping a youngster work through them will increase the chances of successful eating.

2. Avoidance responses are acquired through experience: they are adaptive in that they enable an individual to avoid what is perceived to be aversive.

3. When a child discovers that one of his behaviors enables him to avoid what he'd rather not experience, that behavior will begin to occur more often when he is once again faced with the same situation.

4. Avoidance responses associated with feeding frequently have their inception due to some physical problem associated either with swallowing or digesting. The learned responses often remain long after the physical problems have been rectified. Often, their continuation is maintained unintentionally by parents or support staff who are unaware of how to deal with the responses. Avoidance responses, too, can be unrelated to physical problems. Instead, they can come about as a direct result of the manner in which the parents respond to the child's behaviors. Such happens when noncompliance to parental requests becomes a frequent occurrence.

5. Avoidance responses will usually be related to one of the following:

   a. The child does not wish to eat because he isn't hungry.
   b. The child does not wish to eat because eating causes him physical discomfort.
   c. The child does not wish to eat because of "emotional" associations with previously experienced feeding methods.
   d. The child will not eat because he has learned that non-eating, rather than the opposite, produces desired attention from his primary feeder. The child will not eat because he doesn't like what is offered.

6. Eliminating interfering avoidance responses requires that we first make certain they no longer serve any justifiable purpose (the physical problems likely responsible for their inception have been rectified). Once satisfied, we need to show the child the avoidance responses will no longer work (they will no longer enable him to avoid participating in the eating sequence).

7. We help the child work through the avoidance responses by treating them as though they did not occur.

8. As we help the youngster relinquish the avoidance responses, we provide him with many alternatively more desirable ways of achieving what he values. Eating and swallowing produce outcomes to the child's liking.

9. During the process that teaches the child his avoidance responses are no longer necessary, the therapist must make certain that the feeding session ends on a positive note. Such an outcome shows the child that feeding can be enjoyable; that his desired responses of cooperation will end the session; and that the following session will be equally enjoyable.

10. Care must be taken to ensure that time constraints do not interfere with the reduction of the avoidance responses. The therapist/feeder must give the child as much time as is necessary to work through each avoidance response. If the therapist believes time will be a problem, the attempted elimination of an avoidance response, particularly one that has existed for some time, would be best avoided until the time factor can itself be eliminated. If the therapist is forced to end a session prematurely while working through an avoidance response, the professional should end the session as quickly as possible. Then, the same therapist, under the same conditions of location, utensils, and foods, must work through the avoidance responses as quickly as possible—preferably the same day.

CHAPTER SIX

The Acquisition and Maintenance Phases

If the exploration phase went well, the therapist/feeder was able to determine:

1. At what level in the eating sequence the child succeeded;
2. The type of artificial reinforcement that appeared to be of value to the child; and
3. The types of avoidance responses the child was most likely to manifest.

As we turn our attention to the acquisition phase, where the therapist builds on the information obtained during exploration, and now seeks to help the child acquire more appropriate and desired eating skills, the above three issues continue to be very important.

Acquisition

The Level at which the Child Succeeds

The acquisition phase is where the therapist will introduce the child to the process that will provide the two most basic components of "po" feeding: the teaching (or reteaching) of the relationship between swallowing and reduction of hunger, and the major contingency that nice things happen when food is eaten by mouth. As introduced earlier, for these two components to be learned, the therapist must begin his or her teaching at a point where the child's success is nearly guaranteed, and the professional must have available something the child values that can be provided when the youngster complies with the therapist's requests. Remember that the child, through her behavior, will tell the therapist/feeder where within the eating sequence success is probable and what will presently motivate her.

NICKI

Notice the importance of determining where along some mentally pictured eating sequence a child will likely succeed. Additionally, note how important it is to have available something the child values that can be used as part of a reinforcement contingency. Notice also how helpful it can be to remind the child of the contingency. These issues increase the likelihood the child will be more successful with "po" feeds.

It had been nearly 2 months since I had last seen the bright, highly verbal 3-year-old child. At that time, she had become a total food refuser due mostly to painful oral treatments for mouth and tongue sores. When I first worked with her, I needed several sessions just to get her to touch an empty cup. The feat was accomplished mostly by insistence. The child's cognitive skills were sufficient for her to realize that touching an empty cup was not capable of producing any physical discomfort. Both of us realized that the cup was quite capable of producing emotional discomfort due to its association with the oral treatments. Six brief sessions (roughly 10 minutes each) were required before the child took her first sip of water from a medicine cup. My insistence was no longer sufficient to motivate the youngster to place water on her tongue. When the set of sessions began where the goal was drinking a few drops of water, the child was watching a tape of Steven Spielberg's *ET*. She was told that she would have to forfeit [temporarily] watching the movie if she failed to allow a drop of water to touch her tongue. Her protests were brief once she realized I was not going to waver. No doubt my neutral position played an important role with helping her go beyond simply touching the cup. Additionally, the requirement literally was that she allow one drop to touch her tongue. Once she took the one drop, I thanked her, told her that she had done well, then I left her hospital room for roughly 30 seconds. "One more drop," I said to her the moment I returned. Upon its successful completion, I again left the room. Notice, she was able to get me away from her by drinking the water. At that point in the treatment, that contingency was fine. Six additional sessions, over two days, were required before a drop of soup and small piece of Jello were tasted. Soon after, the child began to enjoy many miniscule tastes of the food she had once eaten with great zeal. Gradually, her "po" consumption increased. She even looked forward to seeing me. I think she was proud of her own progress and wanted me to know about it.

I received the phone call from Nicki's mother 2 months later. A new problem had surfaced: the child had begun to experience severe stomach pains that were associated with a long-standing physiological problem. Due to the pain, the child began to reduce her "po" feedings. She was returned to the hospital, where her condition could be monitored more closely. Her voluntary food intake had nearly vanished—a situation that only served to increase the stomach inflammation. Liquid medication had been provided that would help the stomach heal itself and significantly reduce the pain. Nicki, however, refused steadfastly to drink the liquid. To get the medication into her, the staff had to hold the struggling child down on her bed, pour the small quantity (5 ccs— 1/6th of an ounce) of medicine into her mouth, and pinch her nostrils shut. Everyone, including the child, rapidly became upset with the method. The child was sent home, and her parents were told to do what they could to get the youngster to drink the medication (that had to be taken, or forced, four times a day).

I met with the child in the kitchen of her home. Reluctantly, she had agreed to stop watching TV in order to be with me. (Her expression, when I first walked into the house, reflected her feelings that she was not thrilled by my presence. I reacted to her as though the opposite were the case. I told her how great she looked and how I enjoyed seeing her again.) While she remained downstairs watching TV, I placed two empty medicine cups on the kitchen table. Behind the cups, rested two syringes: one filled with water, the other containing about 7 ccs of the needed medication. When Nicki first sat down with me, she smiled and showed me how the hair on her head was growing. (She had lost all of her hair when receiving chemotherapy.) As soon as she saw the syringes, however, her face grew very long and she began to cry and whine for her mother who was waiting in another room. (I had already logged in my mind that TV might be a reinforcer I could use. Now, Nicki had provided me with an additional one: the presence of Mom.) "Do you want your Mom here with us?" I asked, investigating whether Mom's presence was an event strong enough to motivate the apprehensive child.

"Yes," she said while crying softly. (The child had told me what she valued at the moment: I had the reinforcement component of the contingency. Next, I had to decide what the child would need to do in order to earn the reinforcer. While I could have chosen most any behavior within the sequence I was picturing in my mind, including swallowing the medicine, I wanted the child to experience success; to realize that she could trust me; that I was going to make this situation as pleasant as possible; and that I was not going to hold her down and force her to do anything. I also wanted her to realize that I was in control of the situation: that to get what she wanted, she would have to do something for me first.)

"Okay, quiet down, stop your crying, and I'll get your mom," I said to her clearly, but gently. The child grew quiet and as promised I brought her mom to the kitchen table. "Do you feel okay now?" I asked the child as she looked toward her mother.

"Yes," she whispered, still very uncertain of what I was going to do. (Since I had not seen her for a long while, I wanted to test her "comfort" zone regarding the cups, swallowing, and the liquids.) "I'm glad. This isn't going to be bad. I promise you, no one is going to hold you down or force you to drink anything. Okay?" She nodded. "What I'd like for you to do is to pick up one of the medicine cups and pretend there's water in it. Bring it to your lips and pretend to take a big swallow." She smiled at me, probably remembering that was the approach I first used with her months earlier. She complied with ease. "Water taste good?" I joked.

"Pooey," she exclaimed, a smile now covering her face.

"Okay, now watch what I'm going to do." I lifted the syringe of water and placed about 5 ccs into the medicine cup. Nicki began to whimper. (It was an avoidance behavior—one most understandable given her recent experiences at the hospital.) "Now relax," I urged. "It's just water."

"But I don't want any," she cried.

My face grew a little more firm: "Do you want your mom to stay with us?" She nodded yes. "Then please do as I ask: lift the cup and place one drop of water on your tongue. One drop! Don't drink it," I said, hoping to produce a smile. She complied. "Wasn't bad, was it?" I asked her.

"No," she said with a whisper.

"Well, you did great. Okay, let's try that once more. Two drops this time, okay?" She took the two drops easily. (It was apparent that drinking water from a cup was not going to be much of a problem. It was now necessary to see how far she would go with the medication.) As soon as I lifted the syringe housing the medication, Nicki began crying once again. (Again, an understandable avoidance behavior.) "It's okay, dear, I'm just going to put some of this stuff into the cup. No big deal," I said to her as nonchalantly as possible. (I put about 2 ccs of medicine in the cup.) I moved the cup next to the one with the water, then I sat back in my chair. I explained to her why the medication was necessary; I promised her that no one was going to hold her down; I purposely asked her if she enjoyed being held down at the hospital (her offered "no" was emphatic); then I reassured her that nothing like that would happen. "Here's what I want you to do for me: I want you to pick up the cup with the medicine. Don't drink it, just pick it up." She hesitated; I pushed a little. "Nicki, come on now, this is no big deal. Just touch the cup and pick it up. You don't have to drink it, yet." She reached for the cup and lifted it an inch or so off the table. "Good, now put it down," I said to her. "How was that? Did it hurt?"

"No," she replied.

"Well, you're doing great. I'll bet your mom's proud of you. Why don't you ask her?"

Nicki turned to her mom: "Are you proud?" the youngster asked.

"Yes," her mother responded enthusiastically. "I think you're doing super," the woman added.

"Okay, Nicki, real quick now, do that once more for me: lift the cup off the table." (Up to this point, I hadn't needed to rely on the available reinforcement, but the logical flow was about to reach a level where watching TV was probably going to be necessary.) "Okay, sweetheart, now do this for me," I said, my voice very lively. "I want you to lift the cup and have it touch your lips. Now do it real quick. That's it," I verbally supported as she took the cup of medicine and touched it to her lips. "Okay, now take the cup of water and put a drop of water on your tongue, you know, like you did before." She did it without hesitation. (Notice how I used the agreeable water as a reinforcer for the less agreeable medicine. The eventual contingency: a drop of medicine, a drop of water.) "Now, real quick," I said with animation, "grab that other cup and put a drop of medicine on your tongue. Just one drop. Then take a drop of water and put it on your tongue." I moved closer to her to make sure that one drop of medicine landed on her tongue. When it did, she took at quick drink of water. "Fantastic," I exclaimed. "Do you know what you did?" I asked. "Do you?" I repeated with enthusiasm.

"I took some medicine," she said proudly.

"Right," I applauded. "You took some medicine. Now, real quick, do it again for me. One drop of medicine, then one drop of water. " After she repeated the above request the third time, the medication (the 2 ccs) had been consumed. "You did fantastic," I said to her as I took the syringe and placed another 3 ccs of medicine in the cup. "Hey, I've got a great idea. How would you like to go downstairs and watch TV?" I asked her, as I was about to present the full contingency. She nodded "yes," happily. "Okay, real quick now, finish what's in that cup and then go downstairs and have a good time with the TV." Her face lost a slight touch of its previous joy. (The 3 ccs probably looked to her to be nearer a gallon.) I tried to "catch" her quickly, restating the contingency, assuring her the task was "easy": "Just drink that little bit, then you can go downstairs. You want to watch TV, don't you? Good," I responded when she nodded, "then do this real quick." She took it in one mouthful, swallowed some water, climbed out of her chair and ran downstairs. Her mother and I reviewed what had happened.

"I didn't realize how important it was to have her do something first, then get something she would prefer," the mother said.

"It is essential that Nicki see some reason for doing what is being asked. If she can understand that something pleasant will happen after she has done what you've asked, she will be more inclined to cooperate. I need to try one more thing, " I said to the woman, as I poured 2 ccs more of the medication into the cup. "I want you to take this downstairs, tell Nicki that I goofed, that I didn't have her drink enough, and that she needs to drink this little bit. Notice," I said to the mother, "the TV will be on. If Nicki refuses, restate the contingency: drink your medication and you can watch TV." The contingency was not necessary. Nicki took the cup and swallowed the medication. She smiled broadly. "Would you like to throw that cup into the garbage?" I asked the youngster.

"Yeah!" she exclaimed. Mother brought a trash basket into the room and the child exuberantly slammed the empty cup into the bottom of the basket.

I looked toward the child: "You will have to take some more medication later today," I said to her, "and as soon as you finish it, make sure you take that cup and throw it way!" The assurance was clearly visible across her face.

The "This First" Contingency

As was evident in Nicki's case, each reinforcement contingency required that the child do something first before receiving what she desired. Such a relationship between the needed behavior and the reinforcer can be communicated either through words: "Do this first, then you may have this," or through actions: the child is given a small spoonful of baby fruits followed immediately by a small spoonful of a more preferred food or drink. (Recall that a contingency is simply a relationship between behavior and environmental feedback. Grandma's Rule incorporates contingencies: "Eat your peas [requested behavior] and you can have a piece of pie [offered environmental feedback]," and the procedure of shaping [reinforcing small steps toward a goal] uses contingencies to help the child move "up" the ladder toward the goal.)

During the acquisition phase, where I am trying to teach a child any number of important lessons regarding feeding, I always try to have a valued object that will allow me to practice the concept of "this first, then this." Most times, I will hold the desired object up to the child and take a spoonful of food or cup of liquid and present that to the child. Then I will ask, "Do you want *this*?" emphasizing the valued object. When the child says yes (or nods), I will explain, "This first," bringing the spoon into the child's mouth, "then this," immediately handing him the object he wanted. After a few seconds of playtime with the valued object (which could be listening to music, looking in a mirror, listening to a story, etc.) I will remove it from the child, refill the spoon, place the food into the child's mouth, followed again by handing him what he wants. Throughout the exercise I always repeat, "This first," when giving the child the food, "then this," when giving him what he wants.

This same "this first" approach is equally important and effective with older children whose goals will likely refer to broadening food choices or complying with a parent's request to finish a portion of a particular food. Again, identification of a valued object, activity, or food is given to the child after she complies with the parent's request to try a small amount of a new food or finish what was requested. The older child's language skills allow the therapist/feeder and child to verbally practice the precise elements of the "this first" contingency. The child can be requested to state precisely what she must do in order to gain access to what is desired.

"Going Through" Avoidance Responses

When the child is faced with the "this first" requirement, the stage is set for the occurrence of avoidance responses. Nicki's avoidance behaviors were primarily verbal accompanied by some crying. Regardless of what they were, they would not have been allowed to either end the session or result in the child gaining access to what she preferred. For a child to receive what she desires, the "this first" component must be complied with.

Occasionally, what was once valued by the child may become quite meaningless, given the fact that the youngster now has to do something to receive what she initially desired. "I don't want to play with the bear, or go outside" the child might say through words or actions. (Nicki might have said that she didn't want to watch TV.) Under such conditions, the therapist/feeder will need to identify something else the child might be willing to work for. Determining the potentially valued alternative often is not easy. Often the only thing the child wants is for the session to end. Great. There's the reinforcing component of the contingency: "As soon as you swallow (or whatever response is guaranteed to be something the child can do), we're finished."

A Mini-Review

Think of the three factors we have covered so far.

1. Start at the level where the child can succeed.
2. Identify reinforcers, and use a "this first" approach with the youngster.
3. Be willing to go through the manifested avoidance responses.

Stay with the above factors, and the acquisition phase will be moving in the right direction.

Process More Important Than Quantity

By remembering the two basic components that will be taught in the acquisition phase:

1. The teaching (or reteaching) of the relationship between swallowing and reduction of hunger, and
2. Nice things happen when food is eaten by mouth,

it will be easier to understand why learning the process involved with "po" feeding or broadening a diet is initially much more important than the quantity of food that is consumed. With the above in mind, consider the following suggestions.

Food Selection during Acquisition Phase

Excluding some unusual medical justification to the contrary, nutrition, at first, is less important than practicing the relationship between swallowing, reduction of hunger, and artificial reinforcement. Check with the child's attending physician to see if any specific foods are "out." (Some children have food allergies, thus the child's sensitivity to certain foods must be considered.) During the beginning part of this phase, select the easiest, favorite foods. If, as may happen with infants and slightly older youngsters, favorites and "easy ones" are a mystery, go with some simple pudding, yogurt, baby cereals, fruits, juices, or plain or flavored milk. Again, the foods are simply a vehicle to help the child learn the process. Remember, during the acquisition period, the therapist's sole intent is to teach the child that he can reduce hunger and gain lots of positive feedback by consuming things by mouth. There will be plenty of time, once the process of "po" eating has been acquired, to alter diets in any way the family physician and dietitian believe is appropriate.

If the therapist/feeder is working with a very young child, and is uncertain about which foods to use, the professional might consider the following: if the child has been fed exclusively (or nearly so) with liquid formula, try using solids (baby cereals mixed with strained fruits) during the acquisition period. Or, if the child's foods have been primarily solids, try using primarily liquids. Several of the infants seen were quickly helped by giving them practice with cereals (followed by drinks of formula) rather than formula alone. The youngsters seemed to experience less difficulty moving the cereal around in their mouths, thus giving them more control with the food which, in turn, may have helped them to feel less fearful. After only a handful of sessions, the children began to eat more readily, perhaps because they learned that their hunger was satisfied by swallowing the cereal.

Multiple, Brief Sessions

For the duration of the acquisition phase, the therapist will want to provide the child with many brief opportunities to practice the contingencies being used, and will want the child to experience the professional's determination to "go through" the previously successful avoidance responses. *The more sessions the feeder provides, spread throughout the day, the greater the chances the child will learn and retain what has been taught to him.* Sessions that are brief increase the likelihood that both the therapist/feeder and the child will experience greater pleasure and less frustration. From the child's perspective, the brief sessions may be a welcome relief from what he has been experiencing.

While there are no absolute guidelines regarding time per session, and sessions per day, I have found the following sequence to be beneficial:

1. During the first few days when I am trying to help the child understand the benefits and processes involved in eating by mouth, I try to have at least five or six sessions per day, each one lasting no more than 10 to 15 minutes.
2. As progress is observed, the sessions per day decrease, and time per feeding increases according to the child's caloric consumption.

Several issues are involved with this alteration of time and sessions per day. Ideally, the therapist will want to make sure the child is somewhat hungry prior to the next meal. The child's ability to maintain a feeling of hunger may be the deciding variable when determining how many sessions are feasible throughout the day.

The actual length of each session cannot be completely fixed, although again, they initially need to be brief. The child's performance during a session ultimately determines that session's length. By remembering that it is absolutely essential that each session end on a positive note, it becomes apparent why the time period of any given session will be variable. Regardless of the minutes involved in the session, the therapist wants the child to experience pure success with the process of eating by mouth. That's the goal. The feeder may find, during the first or second session of the acquisition period, that a 3- or 4-minute session is perfect: the child has tried a few things and has succeeded. A later session may require 6 minutes before the professional believes an important lesson has been learned. Again, time, *per se*, is not the issue; what the child does during the time period is the crucial component.

Successful Sessions

The more successful sessions the child experiences, no matter how brief their duration, the sooner the child's "po" feeding will come under the control of natural feedback. During each session of the acquisition phase, therefore, every effort is made to have the child experience preferably all, but certainly some, of the following:

1. A reduction of hunger by "po" feeds.
2. Pleasant tastes.
3. A weakening of avoidance responses.
4. A decrease in any fearful associations with "po" feeds.

As is evident, process is much more important than the initial quantity of food that is consumed. Five successful small bites, where each of the above four components is experienced, is infinitely more valuable than the consumption of 50 bites, where none of the above has been experienced (excluding perhaps number 1, which may have been achieved through unpleasant means). The feeder wants the child to learn that nice things happen when he eats by mouth. The more often the child learns that, the more rapidly the youngster will understand the relationship between swallowing and reduction of hunger.

Shaping

The "art" and "science" of this process to help the child eat by mouth rests, in part, on the therapist's ability to guide the child gradually from his level of successful eating to the level that is desired for him. When I begin working with the child during this acquisition period, my intent is to take the child from wherever he is and move him gradually, comfortably, successfully toward the next sequential step. The following "schema" has become a permanent part of my thinking as I try to determine what experiences or exercises might help make the child's learning easier. Frankly, the process of shaping is not something that can be taught effectively by reading a few passages in a book. The learning requires hands-on experiences, often with supervision. Nevertheless, I'd like to present this schema (or model). It might offer a way to view the task of taking the child from his successful eating level to a subsequent step, eventually leading to "po" feeding. The model represents the "mentally pictured sequence" referred to during Nicki's case. I knew what I wanted her to do; I found out what she was willing to do; then I pictured a bridge that would connect the two points together. The bridge became the mentally seen sequence:

Goal: "Po" eating

7

6

5

Steps (the bridge): 4

3

2

1

Present Performance Level

The goal, of course, represents what the therapist/feeder wants the child to do: eat or drink by mouth, consume greater quantities of food, try or finish foods. The "Present Performance Level" represents what the child is presently doing: the eating level at which he presently succeeds and the level at which the avoidance behaviors begin to show themselves. The word "Steps" represents the experiences and exercises the professional will use to help the child move from where he is to where the therapist would like him to be (in other words, move across the bridge or "up the ladder"). These experiences and exercises represent the heart of the shaping process. Let me offer a quick, practical example of how the above model can be used.

NANCY

Notice how the components of the above model are sequentially considered and employed during the exploration/acquisition phases. Note the term "error analysis" that will be introduced. Eventually, the term and the operations it represents will be critical parts of the therapist's thinking as he or she sets about to help a child progress through an eating sequence.

The 2-year-old had been brought in from out of state in order to have her eating behavior evaluated. After an extensive interview with the child's parents and attending physician, the goal of "po" feeds producing consumption of 1,000 calories per day was established. (Drinking was not a problem for the child.) The youngster was taken into an examination room at the hospital for the exploration phase.

During the exploration phase, the child's present performance level (the level at which she succeeded, and the level at which her avoidance behaviors became apparent) was determined. The present performance level assessment showed that the child sat comfortably in the high chair and played with a stuffed animal and toy pony that she had brought from home. She was receptive to an empty spoon as it touched her cheek, nose, lips, and tongue. However, when the spoon was one-quarter filled with a type of pudding she purportedly had eaten in the past, she gently raised her head and turned it away to her right. When the spoon was brought to the tray, her gaze returned to the animals she held in her hands.

The exploration process stopped long enough to allow an initial error analysis of the present performance level observations. As the name implies, an *error analysis* is a process that attempts to determine why a child's desired eating behavior stops at a particular point on an eating sequence. Why, for example, did Nancy readily accept an empty spoon as it touched her lips, but work to avoid the one-quarter filled spoon before it reached her lips? The observations were clear: an empty spoon placed on her tongue was no problem; a partially filled spoon created difficulty. Why? Error analysis is a brainstorming exercise that requires that we look at any and all information that might explain both why the desired behavior breaks down as well as what methods or experiences might help the child move beyond that point. In Nancy's situation, the following was known:

1. The child had been kept off food for some 6 hours; chances were good that she was experiencing some degree of hunger.
2. She had a long history with food refusal; augmentative feedings through g-tube had been employed since the child was 6 months old.
3. As a result of her experiences with augmentative feeds, the likelihood was slim that she had any understanding of the concept that swallowing by mouth somehow resulted in the reduction of body hunger.
4. Mother's information had clearly indicated that few, if any, attempts with contingencies involving any sort of feeding and subsequent reinforcement had been made over the past months. Mother further indicated that Nancy could end the "po" feeding sessions by indicating (through body movements) that she was no longer interested in eating or having anything near her mouth. Mother pointed out that she rarely persisted when trying to feed her daughter.

My sense was that I first needed to help the child understand the purpose for eating by mouth. For this understanding to occur, the child would have to increase the occurrences of swallowing food. I realized, however, that swallowing food held little value for her: her feelings of hunger had been satisfied without any active, personal participation; her hunger had been removed through someone else's efforts (her mother's initiated tube feeding). Indeed, the very presence of food as it approached the mouth probably was aversive to the child, hence the reason why she worked hard to avoid it. I believed, however, that I might be able to use the stuffed animal or the toy pony as a means to help the process of swallowing get started. I decided to shoot for the following target behavior: Nancy allowing small amounts of food to be placed on her tongue without manifesting any avoidance responses. I would use a shaping process to help both of us achieve that goal.

I sat in front of her and spoke quietly of the fun we were going to have as I opened a jar of banana pudding. The toy pony and stuffed animal stood on the tray. I wanted Nancy to experience the first of several exercises and contingencies I was going to use. I handed her the toy pony; she eagerly grabbed it and brought it to the side of her face. I picked up an empty spoon and as I gently, but firmly, took the toy pony from her hand, I quietly said, "My turn." Without delay I brought the empty spoon into her mouth, touched it to her tongue, and immediately handed her the toy pony, saying, "Your turn." (Had she not allowed me to place the spoon on her tongue, I would have brought it to her lips, then handed her the toy pony.) I allowed her to play with the pony for 5 seconds. As my hand approached the pony I repeated, "My turn," took the pony in my hand, brought the empty spoon to her tongue, and instantly handed her the animal, saying, "Your turn." I repeated the above sequence three additional times. On each of those trials I held the empty spoon upside down. As the child played with the pony I placed a small amount of pudding on the spoon, turned the utensil upside down, gently removed the toy from the child's hand, saying, "My turn," brought the inverted spoon to the child's mouth, dropped the pudding on her tongue, and immediately handed her the pony, softly saying, "Your turn." (Her reaction was not critical—she could have done whatever she wished, but I was prepared to continue the sequence that I had begun. Happily, Nancy swallowed the pudding.) She was allowed to play with the pony for a few seconds. I removed it with a "My turn," placed a small amount of pudding from the still inverted spoon on her tongue, gave her the toy, saying, "Your turn." After another replication, I turned the spoon rightside up, held the toy, put the spoon and food into her mouth, gave her the toy, and told her how marvelous she was doing. I instituted three more repetitions, then stopped the session, taking her out of the high chair. She was returned to her mother. An hour later, the sequence was repeated 10 times before the session ended. A further session was held later in the afternoon, the particulars being basically the same. The only difference was a gradual increasing of the amount of pudding placed into the child's mouth. With each repetition, the child became more astute at predicting the involved steps: she began to hand me the pony, open her mouth, then hold out her fingers for the toy. On the following day, sweet potatoes were added to the menu. The spoon was no longer inverted as it alternately provided pudding and potatoes to the child. By midday of the second day, Mother had observed enough to take over the contingency and eating sequence. The child manifested an avoidance response the first time Mother brought the spoon toward the child's mouth. Mother caught her child's eyes: "This first," she said firmly, gesturing toward the spoon, "then this," she added holding up the pony. Without delay, Mother placed the spoon into the child's mouth, handed her the pony, and said, "Great eating." Thereafter, the avoidance behaviors stopped.

As may have been evident from the above, shaping is simply a process that tries to find subtle ways of making complex problems easier to achieve. It is a process that helps to bridge the gaps that exist between where a child succeeds and where the youngster stumbles. It takes the child from some point and helps her move up the ladder. I knew from the exploration phase that Nancy had no problem with an empty spoon. While I recognized she wasn't thrilled about a spoon partially filled with food, I also realized that she wasn't aware that nice things could happen if she would swallow what was provided. Turning the spoon upside down allowed me to introduce her to a positive, artificial consequence that otherwise might have required a power struggle. The simple turning of the spoon made the struggle just a little easier.

Whenever the therapist/feeder is faced with a hurdle that must be jumped, consider the following:

1. Identify the goal needed for the child to achieve;
2. Determine the youngster's present performance level—the level where she succeeds and the point at which the avoidance behaviors begin;
3. Run a thorough error analysis to see if it can be determined what may be responsible for the present avoidance responses;
4. Invent some shortcut, some half-way exercise, some little experience like a twisted spoon or a drop of liquid delivered through a Brecht feeder, or any ingenious step that will make the process of "po" feeding easier. These ingenious steps are limited only by the therapist/feeder's own creativity.

Stabilize the Process

The acquisition period's purpose is to get the process of eating by mouth started on the right foot. Specifically, we try to teach the child gradually, through brief, multiple sessions, using small sips or bites, that nice things happen when food is swallowed by mouth. Quantity is not important, not initially at least. Time is on our side, patience our needed ally. (Patience, sometimes, is hard to come by when it appears as though everything we've tried has failed to move the child closer to our goals. What often maintains my efforts is the knowledge that the child, through his actions, actually is trying to tell me what I need to do in order to succeed. Unhurriedly, I keep plugging away knowing that eventually I, or one of my colleagues, will understand the child's message.)

Whether the youngster has gained the skill of overt speech or whether he is presently limited to private thoughts, we want the child to say to himself "when I eat, nice things happen"; "when I swallow food, my hunger goes away." More correctly, we want the child to accurately describe the precise steps he must take in order to receive both artificial and natural feedback. The more the child experiences the relationship between swallowing and pleasant tastes, swallowing and reduction of hunger, the quicker tubes and consultants will no longer be needed.

Maintenance

By the conclusion of the exploration/acquisition phases, only two of all the children seen (both nearly 2 years of age, both developmentally delayed) failed to show satisfactory improvement in "po" feeding. The children had been augmentatively fed from near birth, and thus neither had ever experienced any ownership of the process that produces a reduction in hunger from swallowing. Their "po" eating continued to be insufficient to maintain growth, thus requiring continuation of g-tube feedings. The rest of the children did well during the early phases. ("Well" means they experienced, to some degree, all of the following):

1. A reduction of hunger by "po" feeds.
2. Pleasant tastes.
3. A weakening of avoidance responses.
4. A decrease in any fearful associations with "po" feeds.

Once a youngster began to eat by mouth, eat more varied foods, or finish what was expected of him, it was necessary to move to the critical second stage: maintaining the newly or reacquired eating behaviors, and helping the parents take over (or continue with) the responsibility of feeding their child. Both goals are essential, of course, otherwise whatever gains are made during exploration/acquisition will be of little value.

To begin the discussion on maintenance, it is necessary to divide the children into two groups:

1. Those whose eating is totally or partially through an augmentative feeding regime; and
2. Those whose consumption of food is totally by mouth.

Maintaining whatever success has been achieved through exploration and acquisition will differ considerably depending upon these conditions.

Augmentative Feeds as an Ally

When a child is being fed augmentatively, the therapist/feeder is provided with a great deal of flexibility. If "po" methods are not overly successful in terms of quantity, the feeder can always feed and hydrate the youngster in order to maintain his health. Such an advantage, however, presents us all with one of those Catch–22 scenarios: the more we augmentatively feed, the less likely the child will be hungry; the less hunger, the less the child will eat by mouth; the less eating by mouth, the more necessary it becomes to augmentatively feed. As I've indicated several times, when a child is fed through a tube, he learns nothing about the relationship between swallowing and reduction of hunger. If, indeed, a lesson is learned, it is that someone else, somehow, removes the feeling of hunger. Such a lesson does not enhance the acquisition or maintenance of "po" feeding.

While initial acquisition of "po" feeding can be facilitated by careful manipulation of augmentative feeding, maintenance of what has been acquired is totally dependent upon such manipulation. The child must, periodically and predictably, experience a sense of hunger and repeatedly experience the reduction of that hunger by "po" feeding before the natural feedback can maintain eating by mouth. For that to happen, several issues need to be taken into consideration, the most important of which is listed first:

1. Augmentative feeds must not be altered or manipulated in any manner without the full understanding and consent of the child's primary physician.
2. Before augmentative feeds are manipulated significantly in order to increase the child's state of hunger, the child must have experienced several experimental sessions where he

was observed to manifest many successful swallows of food. In other words, the child, through an exploration/acquisition period, must have acquired the skills necessary to eat by mouth. Understatedly, *it is not in the child's best interest to feel suddenly hungry but not know how (or not be able) to alleviate the sensation.*

3. Manipulation of augmentative feeds often takes one of three forms: (a) a gradual reduction of calories per augmentative feed; (b) the elimination of one or two consecutive augmentative feeds, producing a 4- to 8-hour food-deprived period; or (c) a total elimination of augmentative feeds (not including hydration) for a few days. The child's primary physician must decide which of the above approaches, given the child's uniqueness, is most suitable. At the same time, the child will let the therapist/feeder know through his behavior, which of the above approaches will produce the best results. Each of the approaches proved itself to be beneficial with certain of the seen children, although by far the most effective method was "c." It seemed that many of the children required more than 24 hours (often 48 to 72 hours) without food before they began to show some interest in "po" feeding. Again, a critical reminder: withholding of food cannot be considered an available option unless unequivocal data are available showing the child is capable of reliably swallowing by mouth.

In the Absence of Augmentative Feeding

Maintenance of "po" eating, whether accompanied by augmentative means or not, is dependent upon the same three issues we've mentioned so many times:

1. Food swallowed produces pleasant tastes;
2. Food swallowed reduces hunger; and
3. Food swallowed does not result in physiological discomfort.

Thus from a purely physiological viewpoint, maintenance of "po" feeding is not overly complicated. If the above three factors are working in our favor, "po" feeding should occur regardless of which environmental cues are present. At the same time, persistent "po" feeding does not always happen overnight. Frequently, several additional exploratory sessions were needed to evaluate sudden spurts of eating that were followed by sudden refusals to do the same. Some of the children seen required many weeks (some, months) of practice before their frequency of swallows and concomitant weight gain showed a marked, positive acceleration; others progressed rapidly, almost as though an eating problem had never existed. A few of the children required the use of artificial reinforcement for "po" feeding throughout a month or so of maintenance sessions, while most of the children's "po" eating came under the influence of natural feedback quite rapidly. An occasional "this first then this" contingency seemed to help the children remember what they were to do. (While it was difficult to predict how much time and practice would be required before significant gains in "po" eating were manifested, there did appear to be a strong, direct relationship between time and the following two variables: months of required augmentative feeding, and the degree of discomfort the child previously experienced with "po" eating.)

Generalization

It is of course necessary to eliminate the need for neutral feeders and neutral locations, thus allowing parents to maintain full responsibility for their child's eating. To accomplish this generalization from therapist/feeder to parent/feeder, the child's previously manifested avoidance responses, that once occurred in the presence of the parents, have to be reduced to a point where they no longer interfere with "po" feeding. Reduction (or elimination) of avoidance responses are brought about by:

1. Having a neutral feeder show the child the avoidance re-

sponses are no longer necessary and will no longer work; then

2. Having the parent replicate the exact methods employed by the neutral feeder so the parent will no longer be a cue in the presence of which the avoidance responses will occur.

Once I have successfully worked through the child's avoidance responses in a neutral location, I will bring the child's parent into the room where the exploration/acquisition exercises took place. Depending upon the severity of the child's avoidance responses and the time it took to reduce them, I may position the parent many feet from the child or have the parent sit in the chair I previously occupied. (I will use a shaping approach to gradually move the parent physically closer to the child if such a step-by-step process appears warranted.) While there's considerable guesswork involved when attempting to figure out where the parent should first be positioned, I usually suggest that the "softer" the child's avoidance responses, the closer the parent can be to where the child is seated. Occasionally, the child will begin crying, screaming, or thrashing upon first seeing her parent in the room. More times than not, again depending upon the severity of the newly manifested "avoidance" responses, I will ask the parent to leave the room, thus allowing me to work through the child's responses. When the child relaxes, I will bring the parent back into the room.

Eventually, I must have the parent seated in front of the child in a manner very similar to how the parent feeds at home. The purpose for this early generalization phase is to nearly replicate the typical feeding situation the parent will use when feeding the child alone at home. Therefore, I will have the parent sit in front of the child as quickly as possible, and I will stand directly behind the parent. Remaining close by allows me to talk the parent through the procedures, critique the parent's actions, support the parent's efforts, and, if necessary, step in and help the parent if the child's avoidance behaviors unexpectedly resurface. Most of the parents, after only a few minutes of practicing with the employed contingencies, or reminding the child "this first, then this," or maintaining a firm voice while "going through" an avoidance response, assimilated the procedures quickly and naturally and required very little further assistance. Occasionally, a parent would need several practice sessions before demonstrating attention to the determined target behavior and the needed quickness with the contingencies. By and large, generalization in the neutral setting was not much of a problem.

Generalization from the neutral setting to home, however, was often much more difficult. Invariably, the child, once back in familiar settings, surrounded by familiar cues, "tested" the parent's convictions, patience, and skills. The first few meals were always the most critical: if the parent could work through the manifested avoidance responses immediately, they grew weaker rapidly. If, however, the parents, now surrounded by the same familiar cues, became lax and reverted to former feeding methods, the avoidance responses reemerged and were as strong as they had ever been. Therefore, before a parent attempts feeding at home, the therapist/feeder must be completely satisfied that the parent knows precisely what to do when the child eats comfortably, as well as what to do when (or if) the child manifests the previous avoidance responses. A little extra practice with the parent and child alone in a neutral setting often makes the return to home a little easier and more successful. If the parent feels somewhat insecure about the first "going it alone" session at the house, it can be helpful for the therapist/feeder to accompany the parent and child so as to be close by during that first home feeding.

Generalization from a neutral setting within the home to a nonneutral setting in the home can be the most difficult. It is nearly impossible to achieve a neutral setting within the child's home. Familiar cues that have been associated previously with eating are constantly available. Nevertheless, an approximation to neutrality can be achieved. For this to occur, a location far removed from the previous feeding location needs to be found. In the past, I've used finished basements, hallways, living rooms, and most any other location where the child has had little, or preferably no, previous experiences with eating. The exploration/acquisition sessions occur in this location. Once the child shows an increase in successful swallowing, consideration can be given to moving the feeding sessions back to the more familiar location (e.g., kitchen). If the child's behavior regresses as soon as feeding occurs in that location, then the neutral setting should once again be used. In addition, if there is regression, the feeder (therapist or parent) must check to make sure the child is hungry; he is experiencing pleasant tastes; he's not experiencing any physical discomfort; the feeder is using contingencies correctly; the feeder is not giving in to avoidance responses, as well as considering the many other variables we have discussed. As a reminder of the importance of these "other" factors, if a child is not hungry, location, be it neutral or otherwise, will have little impact on his eating.

Gradual Introduction of Variety

Through exploration, acquisition, and the first several sessions during maintenance and generalization, the process of establishing the relationship between swallowing and reduction of hunger has taken precedence over quantity of food consumed, as well as the variety of foods consumed. Once the child's behavior has begun to come under the influence of natural feedback and she understands what her swallowing produces, a gradual introduction of a variety of foods (and textures) should be considered. Notice, however, the word "gradual." We do not want the child to become frightened by some overwhelmingly foreign object that has suddenly found its way into her mouth. Nor do we want to force a power struggle (particularly if "po" feeding is starting to become a natural part of the child's repertoire) by requiring the child to eat something solely because of its color or vitamin content. Introducing variety and texture needs to be done in a relaxed, casual manner. Patience and a consultation with a dietitian are the best options when desiring to add variety and spice to a child's newly acquired appetite.

Consultation with a Dietitian

There's another reason to have a consultation with a dietitian besides asking questions about variety and spice. These people have a way of taking mundane foods that contain at best a handful of calories and "punching" that stuff into tasty, high-caloric treats (that are healthy, besides). As is obvious, the issue of calories with food-refusal children is important.

Until a child's appetite grows sizably to where consumption of sufficient food is no longer a problem, we will always want feeding time to be brief, not protracted. Brief, from the child's viewpoint, is often much more palatable. But brevity may not produce enough consumption to satisfy a child's growing caloric needs. Ever noticed how many calories there are in a small jar of baby food? Not too many. Enter dietitian (and physician). So long as there are no physiological contraindications, foods for the food refuser should be "punched up" in calories. There are puddings and liquids that contain megacalories per ounce that can be used as supplements to regular foods. There are tasty ways of making baby sweet potatoes, meats, vegetables, and the like, into "caloric" delights so that long sessions where x number of calories have to be consumed can be shortened and still be calorically successful. With a little ingenuity and the help of a professional who knows all the ins and outs of the food groups and how to enhance the caloric value of each, the task of "po" feeding can be less time consuming, more productive, and infinitely more enjoyable for all parties involved. So important is the dietitian to the goal of helping the food refuser consume nutritional calories, one who will talk about "punching up" foods and lots of other important topics will join us shortly.

Summary

1. Once completing the first phase of exploration, the therapist/feeder should have some sense of where the child succeeded on the eating sequence; what type of reinforcement might be valued by the youngster; and what types of avoidance responses might be expected during future feeding sessions.

2. During acquisition, the feeder will want the child to begin to learn that she, not someone else, can bring about a reduction of her gnawing hunger; that through some active, personal response—swallowing—not only will the hunger dissipate, but other nice things will also happen.

3. Often the use of reinforcement contingencies, where the child is required to manifest a behavior before receiving what she values, is an optimal vehicle that will begin to teach the child she can actively satisfy her own hunger drive.

4. When using contingencies, make certain the child has the necessary skills to succeed and thus gain access to the reinforcers being offered.

5. When working with a verbal child, restating the contingency with mention of the reinforcer first, can help the child understand what she must do to earn what she wishes. The verbal child can also be requested to repeat the precise "this first" contingency, thereby allowing the therapist/feeder or parent to know if the child is aware of what she must do to gain access to the reinforcer. The nonverbal child (as young as 1 week of age) will learn the contingency by multiple, precise presentations of the reinforcer immediately after the desired behavior has been manifested.

6. Multiple practice sessions using a "this first" approach will also help the child learn what she must do to gain access to her reinforcers.

7. During the learning of the contingencies, avoidance responses must not be allowed to interrupt the lessons being taught. The child must learn that her avoidance responses will not get her what she desires.

8. When first teaching the child that her swallowing of food will result in pleasant outcomes, type or quantity of food is not critical.

The process involved with eating and its outcome are the essential lessons being taught. By using multiple, brief sessions, where the child can continuously and frequently experience success, the lessons being taught will be more quickly learned and permanently remembered. As guidelines, consider the following:

   a. During the first few days in the acquisition phase, try to have at least five or six sessions per day, each one lasting no more than 10 to 15 minutes. (A session can be extended if the child suddenly shows great interest in eating. At the same time, the therapist/feeder needs to end the extended session on a positive note.)
   b. As progress is observed, the sessions per day decrease and time per feeding increases according to the child's caloric consumption.

9. A successful session is defined as one where the child experiences some or all of the following:

   a. A reduction of hunger by "po" feeds.
   b. Pleasant tastes.
   c. A weakening of avoidance responses.
   d. A decrease in any fearful associations with "po" feeds.

Keep in mind that 5 successful small bites, when each of the above four components are experienced, are infinitely more valuable than the consumption of 50 bites when none of the above has been experienced.

10. Shaping involves taking the child from where she can succeed (her present performance level) and gradually, successfully moving her further along the eating sequence. It is a process that bridges the gap between where she succeeds and where she begins to falter. The key to successful shaping is represented by the therapist's creative exercises and experiences that will help the child move toward the goal the professional has in mind.

11. Note carefully where the child's successful eating behavior breaks down. Run an error analysis to see what variables appear to be associated with the child's difficulties. Error analysis will lead to those methods that will best facilitate the child's growth.

12. Maintaining the eating behaviors learned during exploration/acquisition requires that the child repeatedly experience the reduction of hunger through her own efforts. For that to occur, of course, the child will need to experience hunger and will need to know how to reduce it.

13. Manipulating feeding schedules to increase hunger drive must always be supervised by an attending physician. This point is essential, for many children will require many hours of no food before they will sense hunger and be willing to work to remove it. Some children, however, due to physical complications, may not be able to tolerate such a length of time without provided nourishment.

14. Generalization of what has been learned through exploration/acquisition is accomplished by having the parent replicate the exact successful methods employed by the neutral feeder.

15. The process of generalization must be done slowly and carefully; the parent must feel comfortable with the methods. Supervision of the parent's efforts is essential, particularly when the child is first taken home, when the child is first being fed by the parent, or when the parent is initiating a new program to broaden the child's diet.

CHAPTER SEVEN

Compliance

All of the children seen manifested some degree of noncompliance: they were requested to swallow food by mouth and, for all purposes, refused. Most of the children's noncompliance and accompanying avoidance responses were so thin, however, that reversing them required little more than patience, persistence, a few words, perhaps a handshake, and an exciting contingency. Several of the children, however, manifested such excessive noncompliance and avoidance behaviors that it was necessary to terminate my exploratory efforts. As indicated earlier, it was apparent within minutes of the initial session that the children's behaviors would not be influenced by ignoring, redirection, verbal explanations, or any available reinforcement contingency. The presence of a spoon, fork, or plate was enough to elicit loud clamoring, thrashing, or gagging. Several of the older verbal children, with defiance written on their faces, flat out exclaimed they would not eat anything. Some, who were seen at home, walked away and locked themselves in their rooms, leaving me with my mouth agape. (Often the parents indicated that the children were equally noncompliant with them, that getting them to follow simple directions or adhere to minimal requests was nearly impossible. Several parents pointed out, prophetically, that getting their children to eat was the least of their problems.)

During the initial meeting with these children, insistence or minimal pressure for them to comply with my requests (or tolerate the presence of a feeding utensil or plate of food) only made matters worse: their expressed avoidance responses became more intense. When time would not allow the opportunity for working through the avoidance responses, the goal for the meeting changed from evaluating where the children were on the eating sequence to ending the sessions on as pleasant a note as possible. On a couple of occasions, "pleasant" translated into trying to help a child calm down so I could get him out of the chair or just say goodbye. Since continued efforts to redirect the children were unlikely to enhance "po" feeding but were very likely to serve the unintended purpose of strengthening the avoidance (and noncompliance) responses, the decision was made to end the sessions as quickly as possible, and provide the parents with suggestions as to how to improve their children's compliance.

Avoidance Behaviors

While purely speculative, it is probable that the children were noncompliant long before they were food refusers. Unintentionally, the children were taught, and therefore acquired, ways of avoiding all sorts of activities not of their choosing: bath time, diaper changes, getting dressed, and going to bed on time were several examples mentioned by the children's parents. For the children, being requested to eat certain foods or certain amounts of foods, like so many other things, was not what they wished to do. They, in different ways, said through words or actions, "No." Either not wishing to push the children too hard perhaps because many of the youngsters had experienced horrible physical problems during their young lives, or perhaps preferring not to become embroiled in an unpleasant scene, the parents dropped or modified their initial requests. The children (those who had experienced severe physical problems as well as those who hadn't) inadvertently learned the same lesson for eating as for bedtime: protest enough (cry, scream, yell, throw, twist and shout, along with other similar actions) and the requests would either be altered, delayed, or eliminated. The children's acquired (avoidance) behaviors, disapproved of, no doubt, by their parents, were nevertheless adaptive: the children simply were doing what was necessary to produce what they valued at the moment. Their behaviors enabled them to avoid what they didn't wish to do. Unfortunately, children rarely understand the different outcomes resulting from working hard to avoid bedtime and working hard to avoid eating. In the first instance, all that's lost is sleep. In the second instance, much more is at stake.

Type-One and Type-Two Requests

While a certain amount of noncompliant behavior is quite typical of children as they progress through their developmental years, these behaviors only become a major concern when they begin to interfere with growth and development. Such is the case when the food-refusing child's behavior is a result of his noncompliant actions. Under that condition, our concern is warranted, and our remediation is needed. Fortunately, compliance problems with young children are not difficult to resolve. Remediation first requires that we understand the differences between the two major types of verbal requests most often made of children by their parents:

Type-One Requests: These are requests made of a child where the youngster has no choice but to comply. There are no ifs, ands or buts: once a type-one request is made, the child must comply; it is a requirement.

Type-Two Requests: These represent requests made of a child where the youngster has a choice as to whether he wishes to comply. Type-twos are more suggestions than requirements.

Since there are no cookbooks available listing which requests "should" be type-ones and type-twos, parents and professionals must determine for themselves which requests must be carried out and which ones will be offered as suggestions, where the children have a choice as to their actions.

Verbal Control

The decision as to which requests are required and which are not is anything but a small issue. Compliance problems begin when parent or child becomes confused as to whether it is necessary for a particular request to be carried out. A simple request is made: "Please put on your jacket; it is very cold outside." Is the request a type-one or type-two? If it's a type-one, the child must comply; if it's a type-two, the child can respond, "No thanks, it's not that cold." Now, suppose the following:

1. Neither parent nor child knew whether the request was a type-one or type-two. Present outcome: at the very least, confusion as to whether compliance was or was not required. Future outcome: the next time the same request is made, the child may or may not comply.
2. The request was intended as a type-two. The child exercised his right to choose. Present outcome: no problem— type-twos do not require compliance. Future outcome: the child will likely assume that all further requests regarding wearing a jacket when informed that "it is cold" are type-twos, thus offering him a choice.
3. The request was intended as a type-one. The child says, "No thanks." That's noncompliance! Type-ones must be abided by. Let's give the parent several options.

Option A. Realizing that he or she has never discussed this business of request types with the child, the parent explains that it is necessary for the jacket to be worn; that the request would not have been made if it were not necessary and important; that requests that must be adhered to, from this day forward, will be known as "type-ones"; that such requests will be portrayed by a certain tone of voice, facial expression, or body position; that it would be advisable for the child to comply; that when compliance has occurred, the parent will be very pleased. The child says, "Thanks for the explanations. Where's the jacket?" The parent responds, "Thanks for doing what I asked. I really appreciate that. It helps me a lot." Present outcome: no problem. Future outcome: (1) child will use parent's voice, face, and body cues to determine the presence of type-ones; (2) the child will begin to appreciate the importance of the parent's words; the child will learn to use the parent's words to help him know what to do; the child will begin to understand that his parent would not have asked him to wear the jacket (or do other things, for that matter) unless he or she really wanted it to be worn; the child's behaviors will come under control of those words; (3) the child will learn that his parent is pleased and appreciative of compliance behavior; (4) future compliance will be more probable, making both parent and child happier.

Option B. Taken aback by the child's forthright refusal, the parent , without further discussion, argument, or expenditure of energy, changes his or her mind. The type-one changes to a type-two. Present outcome: for the child, no problem—he doesn't have to wear the jacket. For the parent, he or she can only hope the kid doesn't catch a cold. Future outcome (bleak): (1) the child has learned that his parent is a wimp; (2) the child has learned that if he doesn't want to do something, just say, "No thanks!" (3) the child has learned that his parent's words aren't particularly important; (4) the parent has lost some influence; (5) the parent has lost a part of his or her ability to guide the child through words; (6) the parent is going to hear the "No thanks," response, through words or actions, more often in the future, perhaps when the parent asks the child to take a bite of food or finish a drop of milk.

Option C. Shocked by the child's forthright refusal, the parent firmly insists the jacket be worn. The child, seeing no reason to comply, repeats his refusal. The parent, now angry, raises his or her voice. The child begins to cry; the parent remains silent; the child begins to scream; the parent remains silent; the child throws himself to the floor, pounds his fists (gently) on the carpet. The parent: "Okay, you don't have to wear your jacket. It's no big deal anyway. It's just a jacket," the parent quietly concludes as he or she slips away, sensing somehow, that something else has also slipped away. Present outcome: the child logs which of his feigned, newly discovered avoidance responses worked and didn't work. He'll try them again in the future. Future outcome: Among the many, three that are crucial. (1) The parent has begun to give up all verbal control over the youngster; (2) generalized noncompliance will increase; (3) the child will begin to understand the value and purpose for avoidance responses, desirable or otherwise. He will use them again.

Parents and Therapists: Check Your Requests

Teaching a child to be compliant requires that the parent (or therapist) check the types of requests being made. If you ask your child to do something and you believe she must comply, then you have presented a type-one request to your child. Your child must comply—no ifs, ands, or buts. If necessary, you must help your child comply. Show her that your words are important; that you would not have asked her to do something if you didn't think it necessary and important! Don't change your mind in midstream (unless circumstances literally prevent you from doing otherwise). Think whether compliance is necessary before you make a request.

"Go Through" the Avoidance Response

Do not allow an avoidance response to interfere with a type-one request. Once the request is made, make sure it is carried out—quickly. If an avoidance response enables your child to have her way, that avoidance response will gain strength and begin to generalize to other settings. The sooner you teach the child that her avoidance responses will not influence your decisions, the sooner the responses will give way to alternatively more desired behaviors. At that point, the responses will be less likely to interfere with feeding.

Practice Type-Ones

To enhance compliance and establish verbal control, spend time during the day practicing a few type-one requests. Select simple activities, those that will create little problem for the child, and have the child do as you ask; specifically, have the child do as you ask as soon as you ask. (Type-one requests should be complied with immediately. If the child procrastinates, your goal for future practice sessions will be to continue with compliance exercises that will now include the demonstrated expectation that the request will be followed when stated.) By practicing them, you provide your child with more opportunities to learn the process involved with compliance, as well as the need to adhere to your request quickly. Ask the child to bring you a book or pencil. Ask her to put her shoes by a chair or her coat in a closet. Ask her to hand you some object or accept some object from you. The tasks aren't too important: they are vehicles for you to practice the whole sequence —the request, the compliance, the demonstrated appreciation (or, perhaps, working through the avoidance responses). The more you practice, the more natural the sequence will fit into your daily routine.

Compliance and Feedback

When a child complies with your requests, two things have actually happened:

1. The child has completed some chore; and
2. She has done what you have asked.

There is a strong possibility that both accomplishments meet with your favor. Since compliance represents behaviors that you would like repeated in the future, it is important to provide the child with some feedback for her efforts. "Thanks for bringing me the book," tells the child that you're pleased that she completed the chore. "Thanks for doing what I asked," tells the child you appreciated her compliance; it tells her that you appreciated the fact that she listened to your words. Never take compliance for granted. Let her know how much you value her attending to your requests. Get her compliance to generalize. By doing so, she might be willing to try some foods on her own. Stranger things have happened.

Develop a Cuing System for Type-Ones and Type-Twos

Because compliance is somewhat dependent upon the child's ability to discriminate type-one requests from type-twos, it is very helpful to provide the child with some cuing system that will facilitate his recognition of whether a request requires compliance. Facial expressions and tone of voice are only two of the ways to help the child with this task. The words you use can also offer a helping hand. Notice the difference in the two requests:

1. "Please put your jacket on."
2. "You can have more meat if you'd like."

How about these?

1. "Bring me the book, dear."
2. "Would you like to go outside?"

There's nothing magical about any of the four statements, but the examples designated by the number "2" seem to be more suggestions then requirements. Experiment with different ways of presenting the requests. You will find a format that makes it easier for your child to understand when he has a choice and when he must do as you have asked. At the same time, watch out for the following:

1. "Would you like to wear your jacket outside?"
2. "Would you like to go to the potty before we leave?"

Anything unusual? They're type-twos, right? Ten bucks to a penny they're disguised type-ones! How many times do you ask your child if he'd like to go to the potty before leaving the house? How many times does he say, "No thanks." How many times do you say, "Sure, let's do it," regardless of what he says. Watch out for disguised type-ones: these are requests that you know your child must comply with, but the child, because of the way you word them, thinks otherwise. It is not only important for the child to believe that your words are powerful, it is also important for him to know that his own have value. If you provide him with a type-two, and he says, "No thanks," his words should be honored. Remember, watch your requests.

Compliance and "Po" Feeding

While it is physically possible to force a child to swallow a few spoonfuls of food or drink a few ccs of liquid, such an approach, of even short duration, will hardly lead to successful "po" feeding, much less pleasant thoughts, feelings, or memories. To a great extent, a child has control over his own eating habits: he can, indeed, keep his mouth shut. Apparent by now, "po" eating will not occur unless the child sees value in the activity: forcing foods rarely produces such vision. One of the major purposes for a therapist's intervention, therefore, is demonstrating to the child that eating by mouth will be followed by pleasant experiences.

The fact remains, however, that a percentage of food-refusing children won't, initially, give therapist or parent a chance to show them the value that comes from eating by mouth: the children manifest severe compliance problems that are secondary to eating. Our task, through assistance offered to parents, is to remediate those compliance issues which, when resolved, will allow us to return to the exploration/acquisition phase with hopes of helping the child eat regularly by mouth.

Again, for the child to eat persistently by mouth, he must experience the three components associated with natural feedback, the components we have mentioned so many times:

1. Reduction of hunger by "po" feeds;
2. Pleasant tastes as a result of "po" feeds; and
3. An absence of physical discomfort as a result of "po" feeds.

If the child's behavior is guided by the above components, acquisition and maintenance of "po" feeding become highly probable.

If, however, the child does not comply with a parent's (or therapist's) request to eat by mouth, his refusal represents his way of telling everyone that something is wrong: he's either not hungry, he's not enjoying what's in his mouth, he's frightened by the eating process, his primary feeders are expecting too much, too soon, or his physical system is providing him with aversive feedback in conjunction with his eating. For compliant "po" eating to occur, these problems must be identified and remediated. The problem is never solely the child's or solely that of the primary feeder. Explaining food-refusal behavior is not that simple.

Influencing Everyday Behaviors

While many problems are mentioned and discussed during the initial interview between therapist and parent, two seem prevalent: providing the food-refusing child attention for *not* eating, and excessive crying that interfered with attempts at "po" feeding. Because these issues are quite common, a word or two about each is in order.

Attention for Not Eating

Inevitably, the food-refusing child will receive a great deal of attention when not eating. Watch yourself for a few meals and note the number of times you request your child to eat or swallow. At the same time, note what she is and isn't doing when you make your request. Attention for not eating is a guarantee. The issue here is not overly complicated: attention can be a motivating variable. To the degree that it is, it can influence the behavior that occurs immediately prior to its application. *Attention provided when the child is not eating can increase not eating! Attention provided for eating can increase its occurrence.* You certainly will want to remind your child (once, maybe twice) of what it is you expect her to do: eat and swallow. However, make certain that your attention, approval, and appreciation occur much more frequently when the child has tasted a food, accepted a spoon filled with new food, or swallowed that which has been provided. As you provide your attention and approval (which, by the way should always accompany the application of other reinforcers for eating, such as music, TV, or whatever your child values), describe to the child exactly what she did that captured your recognition. An exclaimed "Great swallow!" can go a long way toward producing another.

Crying

Also inevitable is a young child's crying. Prior to language development, crying is a major form of communication. Crying, however, that is unrelated to pain or true emotional discomfort, crying that seems more a means to avoid something undesired (like going to bed or having a diaper changed) can begin to interfere with "po" feeding. Crying, of course, can be very difficult to deal with. When it starts to stretch our nerves, we want it to stop. Often, we get it to stop by giving the child what she wanted that started the crying in the first place. Such an approach will only get the crying to stop for the moment. It guarantees the crying will start again before too long. Crying that appears intended to make you change your mind needs to be allowed to run its course—unless you have indeed made a poor choice and thus need to change your mind. Crying that appears intended to allow the child extra minutes of TV or extra ice cream should not be allowed to work. There's no easy way to allow the crying to occur unattended. Some of us read, look at pictures, watch the tube. Others try music or baking. You will need to find an approach that suits your personality. At the same time, recognize that if you occasionally give in to your child's crying, insurmountable problems are not guaranteed, only more crying. Eventually, you will say to your child, "Enough is enough. Go ahead and cry. When you're finished, we'll talk." Until then, you will probably respond to your child's crying as did several of the parents I spoke with during the initial interview. They shared almost identical approaches to dealing with their children's crying, often regardless of what circumstances seemed to set the stage for the crying. All had made the same mistake when dealing with the behavior. The following case will illustrate it.

DONNA

Note which of the child's behaviors helped her gain what she valued.

The 9-month-old's feeding was progressing fairly well. The child's breast feeding was being augmented by recently introduced baby cereals and fruits. Mom's concern regarded a recent reduction in how much food was being consumed. The child's pediatrician had found the youngster to be in excellent health; nothing obvious seemed to be responsible for the slight change in the child's eating. I met with the little girl's mother and asked her to describe a typical scene involving eating. It didn't take long to discover that the child's eating was being influenced by a set of variables not at all uncommon to young parents and their children.

The child was always given the opportunity to sit in her high chair at the dinner table while her parents ate their breakfast and dinner. Finger foods were placed on the tray for the child to do with as she desired, but no demands were made for her to eat. Mother indicated that her daughter generally liked to sit in her high chair at the table for only a few moments; that she preferred to sit in her mother's lap. Mother, on the other hand, had recently chosen for the child to either remain in her own chair or, if she wanted, to play on the floor with her toys. The child would be removed from the high chair when she began fussing and placed on the floor by the table where her toys were located. Invariably, the child would make her way over to her mother, grab her mother's leg, and cry until she was picked up. Mother allowed her child to cry for a few minutes before bringing her into her lap. Once the child quieted, she was placed on the floor. The crying would begin the moment the child was no longer being held. Mother would again ignore the crying for several minutes before taking the child into her arms. The circumstance, however, would soon repeat itself: the child would be placed on the floor; the crying would begin anew; and Mom would pick up the child. Once Mom and Dad became tired of the repetitive scene, the child, upon crying, would be taken to her crib in her own bedroom. Mom would wait about 20 minutes before bringing the still crying child back to the table.

When I asked Mom why she had allowed the child to cry for 20 minutes prior to bringing her out from the bedroom, Mom's response was, "I wanted her to learn that I would not come and get her right away. I wanted her to learn that her crying was not going to work," the young parent added.

Question 1. Which of the child's behaviors most often resulted in her being in her mother's arms? (Answer: The child's crying most often resulted in her being picked up.)

Question 2. What lesson do you think the child learned as a result of the relationship between her behavior and her mother's response? (Answer: Crying increased the chances Mother would hold her in her arms.)

Question 3. What lesson do you think the child learned when having to cry in her room for some 20 minutes before being fetched? (Answer: The child learned that Mom would not come to her right away. The child learned to persist. To keep plugging away. To keep crying, perhaps for as long as twice the amount of time the child was initially left to cry. Despite the fact that Mom wanted her child to learn that crying "was not going to work," Mother's actions taught the child the exact opposite.)

What should Mom do? She and her husband need to decide what they wish their child to do. Sit in the high chair? Play on the floor? Sit in Mom's lap? For the benefit of the child, a decision has to be made. The youngster has little notion of what's going to happen. Once the decision is made, the parents will need to teach their child that a type-one request is in place. The message might be (depending upon the parents' decision): "You can either sit in your high chair, or play on the floor. You can't, however, sit on Mom's lap during eating time. You can sit on Mom's lap at most any other time. Now, if you cry because you wish to be on Mom's lap at the dinner table, you will be placed in your room until your crying stops." Of course, Mom and Dad may decide that it's okay for their child to sit wherever she wishes during dinner. That decision will probably take care of the crying, under the cues of eating time at least.

(In truth, the parents need to decide jointly what they want regarding the entire scope of their child's everyday behaviors. They need to develop guidelines that specify the expectations they have for their youngster's actions. Further, they need to communicate those guidelines to their child. Most of the food-refuser children who had problems with compliance also manifested rather serious problems relating to other activities. The initial interview revealed that the parents had not decided what they wanted their children to do. Behaviors just "sort of happened," often unassociated with rules or consequences. I've met 2- and 3-year-olds who decided what they would wear, when they would sleep, if they would eat, and if their parents were allowed to sleep alone in their bedroom. I've met parents of those children who seemed unable or unwilling to decide whether they wished for their children to have such power. No one, excluding the child, seemed determined to make any decisions about what would transpire within the confines of the family home. Needless to say, progress with "po" feeding rarely occurred until some basic changes regarding compliance, type-one requests, and parental decision-making were observed.)

Summary

1. Generalized noncompliance to daily expectations such as bedtime, diaper changing, and the like, can interfere with the acquisition of "po" feeding.

2. When a child discovers that his fussing allows him to avoid (or delay) bedtime, dressing, or bathing, the youngster may use the same tactic to avoid eating or tasting new, slightly different foods. If such avoidance behaviors work, they will produce problems with feeding.

3. There are two major types of requests that parents use with their children: Type-ones and type-twos.

Type-One Requests: These are requests made of a child where the youngster has no choice but to comply. There are no ifs, ands, or buts: once a type-one request is made, the child must comply.

Type-Two Requests: These represent requests made of a child where the youngster has a choice as to whether he wishes to comply. Type-twos are more suggestions; type-ones are requirements.

Learning the meaning between the two types will help the child comply more readily to parental requests when type-ones are stated.

4. Parents can increase desired verbal control over their youngsters' behaviors by practicing with type-one requests. When doing so, it is imperative that the child carry through with the requests being made and that you acknowledge their compliance. The lesson you want your child to learn is straightforward: show him that your words are important; that you would not have asked him to do something if you didn't think it necessary and important.

5. Be careful of disguised type-one requests—those that you offer as though a suggestion but with which you really want your child to comply. Disguised type-ones need to be avoided. If you wish your child to do something, make certain your words and expressions convey that message.

6. Watch carefully the behaviors that are receiving your valued attention. Responding primarily to your child when he is not eating may interfere with his eating. When he does what you wish, let him know you are pleased. Attend to the desired behaviors he manifests.

7. By allowing a child to cry for 20 minutes and then going to him while he is still crying, you are not reducing the behavior, you are increasing it! If you wish to teach the child that his crying will not bring him what he values, and you have placed him in his room, crib, or playpen, you must leave the child unattended until he is quiet for at least 30 seconds to a minute. The child must learn that his noncrying, quiet behavior will result in your return.

8. It is imperative that you and your spouse decide and agree upon expectations for your child's behaviors. Take paper and pencil and determine what you both want your child to do and not to do. Determine which behaviors will be deemed desired and which will be deemed undesired. Your first step toward teaching your child how to behave is to decide how you wish him to behave. In the absence of that decision the child will determine his own rules and regulations. His decisions may not facilitate his "po" feeding.

CHAPTER EIGHT

Questions and Questions

The uniqueness of each child and the dynamics of the family within which she finds herself guarantee that hitches and glitches will present themselves with our eating programs, despite our best conceived, carefully considered plans and programs. Just when we think we've solved the problem before us, the child offers something new from her side that requires something new from our side. As disappointing (and frustrating) as these unexpected setbacks are, there's always reason and room for optimism. Eating, fortunately, is an activity that carries its own natural feedback. Our task is to figure out how to help that natural feedback work for us and the child.

Over the last several years, while working with the parents of the food-refusal children, numerous questions have surfaced relating to many issues, some directly involving the eating process, others more theoretical in nature. The following is a sample of the questions along with answers based on the past years' experimentations and observations. You will find some of them familiar and perhaps helpful.

1. *If my child has been diagnosed as "failure-to-thrive" (or one who refuses food), does that mean I am a deficient parent?*

Absolutely not! Food refusal can come about for many reasons, none of which necessarily impute responsibility to the primary feeder or caregiver. There are times, of course, when a parent's judgment, which led to significant weight loss in their child, has been less than astute: repeated forgetting to feed a youngster at the prescribed time; a parent limiting her daughter's diet for over a week to a very low caloric liquid, despite being told the child needed 1,100 calories daily; giving in to a youngster's demands for sweets almost to the exclusion of anything else. Such unusual exceptions aside, food refusal can begin under the most innocent of circumstances and grow to immense, serious proportions. The process, occurring right before the parent's eyes, can be quite unrelated to any parental deficiency.

2. *Does food refusal mean the child has a psychological disorder?*

In my judgment, no. Some of my colleagues, however, have differing theoretical views and would likely disagree. They could point to circumstances that in their view would be indicative of a psychological malady or dysfunction. From a practical standpoint, I have no use for either their terms or their theories when it comes to food-refusal children. In fact, I believe that suggesting the child is emotionally or psychologically handicapped diverts our attention from seeing the whole child as an adaptive (nonpathological) individual who through his food refusal is telling us that something is wrong with his physical system or our feeding methods.

3. *What causes "failure-to-thrive" or food refusal?*

More qualified professionals than I have worked on that question since the beginning of the 20th century. Part of the difficulty in arriving at a suitable "etiological" answer rests with the proposed question. *Failure-to-thrive* is a description, not a disease in and of itself. For some professionals, the term represents a symptom of many variables; for others, it is a term that has come to mean more than originally intended; for others still, it is a term that would best be abandoned in favor of something that eliminates the concepts of "failure" and "thrive."

When colleagues have called me seeking assistance with a so-named failure-to-thrive child, I'm reasonably certain I will be seeing a child who is not consuming enough calories by mouth. I don't think of something "causing" the situation in the same way that a physician might say that a germ causes a disease. Instead, I'm fairly sure the child is a food refuser, partial or total. I'm sure that many factors have contributed to the child's present behavior. I'm certain that his food refusing has produced concern among many people.

4. *Okay, so what "causes" the child to be a food refuser?*

Various professionals, discussing the possible causes of food refusal (or failure-to-thrive), believe the "causes" of the condition to be a collective function of the youngster's biological, sociological, and psychological components, as each relates and interacts with the primary feeder's biological, sociological, and psychological components. In other words, no one variable is viewed as totally accountable for the child's food refusal. Let's be somewhat more concrete. Notice the following circumstances and likely outcomes:

a. If the child is not hungry, he will refuse food.
b. If the child doesn't like what's available, he may refuse food.
c. If he hurts when he eats or if he hurts after he has eaten, he will refuse food. If chewing and swallowing require considerable effort, more effort than is judged worthy of the outcome, he may refuse food. If he has discovered that it's a whole lot easier to be satisfied when someone else provides food through a tube, he will refuse food offered at the mouth.
d. If his mother (or father) "forgets" to feed him, he won't be able to eat.
e. If his mother is tired of fighting feeding or if the child is tired of fighting feeding, both may stop (perhaps momentarily) fighting feeding. Maybe Father will help. Maybe Father, too, is tired of fighting feeding; maybe

he's not able to help: the child will refuse food; the parents will refuse to feed. When no one succeeds, it's hard for anyone to keep trying.

Biological, sociological, psychological variables interact with one another in such a way to bring about the child's eating difficulties. Human behavior is rarely simplistic enough to result from a singular, easily discernible cause. You might wish to know that many social scientists have chosen to no longer use the term "cause" when discussing complex human behavior. The term, like so many others, often is interpreted to mean more than intended. Many prefer to speak of variables relating to one another rather than causing one another.

5. *Is it permissible, then, to disregard the "cause(s)" of food refusal?*

It depends upon which "causes" you're referring to. In the "old" days, food refusal was said to be caused by fear of oral impregnation: food was seen as symbolic of sperm, thus food refusing prevented the individual from becoming symbolically pregnant. That kind of a "cause" you don't have to worry about.

Rather than viewing the elements described in answer 4 as causes, it is more helpful to see them as contributing factors to the child's food refusal. A child, for example, might eat a few spoonfuls even though she isn't particularly hungry. She might also eat a little despite the aversive feedback that is experienced while swallowing. These conditions, then, are functionally related to the child's eating: their presence or absence will influence whether the child eats a little or a lot, unpredictably or consistently. The active, functionally related variables that are interfering with "po" feeding must be identified. Once identified, they must be remediated completely. Otherwise, the child may do relatively well in acquisition under a neutral setting but may regress during maintenance at her home. She may eat several bites during one meal, then avoid eating altogether the following meal.

6. *I understand that some children eat fine prior to hospitalization, but often have difficulty eating by mouth during and after the experience. Is that common?*

I don't know how universal such a situation is, but perhaps as many as 15 of the 200 children I saw followed that sequence. They were brought into the hospital for physical concerns unrelated to eating, but after several days of the hospital routine, their "po" feeding came to an abrupt halt. Out of necessity, all of the children required some degree of augmentative feeding, and it appeared that the alteration in the normal feeding sequence, which produced a constant physical sensation of fullness, directly influenced their "po" feeding. Reinstituting "po" feeding was not difficult for over half of the children. Usually several sessions where brief caloric deprivation was combined with some strong contingencies were sufficient to turn the children around. The remaining children, however, required more intensive intervention. By the time I saw them, their avoidance responses had grown in strength. Therefore, in addition to increasing their hunger and establishing strong contingencies, it was necessary to work through their avoidance behaviors.

7. *My child displays very few avoidance behaviors. The one that is most prominent is a tongue thrust which his therapist says is purely volitional, or done by his own choice. He'll do it when he's finished eating, no matter how much or little he's eaten. Have you ever worked with a child who did the same?*

While not questioning your therapist's judgment, it would be advisable to have a second opinion as to the volitional quality of that behavior. If it is indeed volitional, then you will need to treat it like any other avoidance response: you must "go through" it. Place the filled spoon in the child's mouth, press the spoon down on his tongue, and clean the food off the spoon as the utensil is removed. This process tells the child that his response won't work. On the other hand, notice the problem with the above approach if the tongue thrust is not volitional but a function of a neuromuscular difficulty. When looking at any potential "avoidance" response, it is essential to be as certain as possible that the child is capable of controlling the behavior, when and if it occurs. An analysis of the conditions (the cues) under which the "avoidance" behavior does and does not occur can provide you with considerable information about the behavior's volitional quality.

8. *How can you tell if a child's vomiting or gagging is volitional?*

The issues do not change because the behaviors change: we still need to determine whether the child can exercise control over the responses. In the instance of a child's gagging or vomiting, it is absolutely essential that the child be thoroughly examined for physical complications. Simultaneously, the child's behavior should be accurately recorded with specific attention being paid to the conditions under which the behaviors occur and fail to occur. There is an additional consideration that might shed further light on this question of volitional control.

Whenever I view a behavior, any behavior, that is interfering with consistent "po" feeding, I always spend time speculating on the purpose that behavior might be serving for the child. The concept of purpose holds a central theme in the way I view the behavior of children, particularly food-refusing children. My sense is that the child's behavior is not occurring frivolously, capriciously, without intent or purpose. The child's behavior is producing some payoff for her: it is providing her with something that she values. The behavior is either bringing her some reaction that she would like to experience, or the behavior is enabling her to avoid that which she would prefer not to experience. (I recently saw a very bright, articulate 5-year-old who would gag only under very selective cuing situations. Whenever his parents would include vegetables or fruits on his plate he would gag; as soon as the vegetables and fruits were removed, leaving meat and potatoes, he would smile and begin eating. I asked the child why he gagged. He responded, "I don't like those things," pointing to the fruits and vegetables. The child's gagging served a very clear purpose.) When any behavior occurs that appears to be interfering with eating, I will look to see what environmental consequences (or feedback) the behavior is receiving. For example, if vomiting or gagging results in the termination of a feeding session, or if as a direct result of the behaviors the child is removed from what she wishes not to experience, I gain some insight into the possibility that the gagging or vomiting has purpose and intent; thus it is volitional. On the other hand, if the same behaviors occur when feeding is not a present issue, when, let's say, the child is being gently held or is busy playing with toys, I would have a more difficult time suggesting that the behavior held much volitional quality.

Speculating on purpose, then, provides an additional dimension upon which to judge the volitional or organic etiology of a behavior. Together with a thorough physical exam and a carefully documented list of the conditions under which the behaviors occur, we are in a strong position to know whether we will be able to "go through" the interfering behaviors as though they were volitional avoidance responses, or whether remediation will require medical intervention.

9. *Do you recommend telling the child not to gag or vomit?*

Before answering the question, it is necessary first to mention something about conversation during all phases of the eating sequence. Conversation, and the attention that accompanies it, is most often something the child values. It is important, therefore, to attend verbally to the child predominantly when she is either eating successfully or moving in that direction along the eating sequence. As described earlier, asking the child to eat when she is not eating is providing the child with what she values (attention) when she's failing to do what you want. As a general rule, therefore, talk as much as you'd like, as much as you think the child would like. Just remember to talk with the child when she's moving forward; begging her to eat when she's not may move her backward. Now to the question.

Whether the child volitionally gags or vomits, I exercise one of three options. First, I may ignore either behavior or both. If I choose that option, I just allow the behaviors to occur, making no effort to redirect or stop them. Second, I may attempt to stop them through words. "No vomit!" I may state firmly, sharply, the moment the behavior begins. If I choose this response, I will move my body and face closer to the child, often pointing my index finger at her. "No vomit!" I warn, with a serious look on my face. I then watch the child's reaction carefully. (I hope the child is not a projectile vomiter.) If she appeared startled by my reaction and, indeed, attempted to redirect herself once having heard my quick, barbed admonition, I might say in a tone much more pleasant, gentle, and supportive, "Thanks, now let's get back to eating." Third, I may do something I'm not totally comfortable with but have found to produce some interesting reactions. Making certain the child is sitting upright, not leaning back or assuredly not lying down, I may urge the child to vomit or gag! "Go ahead," I may say lightly, leaning back in my chair. "Go ahead, vomit. It's okay. If that's what you want to do, do it. No big deal. I'll clean you up, then we'll start again. Do it," I repeat rather nonchalantly, often using my hands and fingers to signal that I want the behavior to occur. Some of the children who used vomiting to end a session looked at me with total disbelief. If I received that reaction, I urged them more—daring them, almost. From a theoretical standpoint, I did want them to exercise the behavior: I wanted them to see that vomiting was not going to bother me, and it was not going to end the session. A few did regurgitate as requested. They were cleaned, their plate or cup was cleaned, and we both started from square one. Thereafter, they didn't vomit very often. (I would not suggest you employ this third option until you have first discussed it with your child's physician. Depending upon the child's position in a chair, her unique physiology, and the amount of substance she regurgitates, there is a chance for aspiration. Your physician must guide you with this approach. Remember its purpose is to show the child that her volitional vomiting will not be allowed to terminate a feeding session. Given that as the intent, urging the child to vomit is not an essential ingredient.)

You will have to experiment with the above options, and others you might have in mind. I mentioned earlier that I never know ahead of time what I will do with a child. I will try things and watch the youngster's reactions. Her behaviors will tell me if I'm on the right track. Such is the case with how I will react verbally to the child. I'll try one way and watch what the youngster does. Almost always, the child will show me how to reach her.

10. *Is it not acceptable to tell the child to eat or to tell him what will happen if he doesn't eat?*

You can certainly ask the child to eat. In fact, with a kiss to the forehead, you can beg him to eat, once. Just don't ask him 100 times. Once or twice is fine. If he finds out that by not eating you keep talking, and you talk so much that there's no time for eating. . . . More to the point, it is essential that the child know of the contingencies that are operating at the moment. Assuming the child has satisfactory receptive language skills, your words are your strongest suit. But rather than only telling him what will happen if he doesn't eat, remind him once or twice what will happen when he does swallow. In other words, remind the child of the contingency: "As soon as you swallow the fruit, you can have a drink of the milk." Or, "As soon as you finish _____, you can do _____. " Again, once or twice, remind the child of what he's working for: "You want to watch cartoons, don't you? Then, as soon as you _____, you can watch them." Use your words and anything else the child seems impressed by. Just watch when you're interacting with the child. Don't give him a ton of attention when he's not doing what you want.

11. *What happens if you set up a positive contingency and the child, after some private deliberating, informs you that he's not going to do what you want, that he doesn't care about the stupid "reinforcer"?*

One of two situations is probably occurring. First, the payoff may have lost its value—the child has grown tired of watching TV. Second, the payoff may still be very potent, but not potent enough to compete with the child's fear or privately experienced discomfort accompanying eating. If he has grown tired of the original payoff, you'll have to find another. There's nothing magical about this contingency business: without a valued payoff, the desired behavior is not likely to occur. If you will watch the child carefully, listen attentively to his words, he will show you something he values at the moment—something that can be used within a new contingency. On the other hand, if the child's noncompliance is more a function of privately held fears or concerns over possible pain that might occur when he complies with your request, then we have an entirely different situation. Desensitization and shaping may be necessary to help the child with his fears; medical tests may be necessary to uncover why the physical pain is occurring. New contingencies, no matter their value, will not, in and of themselves, be enough if fear and pain are present. They can be a part of the program, but under the above conditions, they can never be the total program.

12. *My child ate so well for her occupational therapist, but as soon as I tried, she reverted to almost total food refusal. Why?*

Assuming nothing unusual happened physiologically, any one of the following is a likely candidate:

  a. The generalization process was poorly designed;
  b. It hadn't been practiced sufficiently to become established;
  c. You didn't work through the child's emerging avoidance responses;
  d. You didn't have a strong contingency available;
  e. You used the contingency incorrectly.

During exploration, acquisition, and maintenance—before the child's eating has come under the control of natural feedback—you must be prepared for a breakdown in the child's behavior whenever feeders, locations, routines, or what have you, change abruptly. The child will test out the new feeder's determination, his or her ability to deal with avoidance responses, and the contingencies that will be in effect. The child can be affected by your consistency, your quickness, your look, manner, or voice.

Make certain, therefore, that the generalization process, incorporating all of the above, has been practiced sufficiently with the neutral feeder close by before you go it on your own. Be prepared for the child's avoidance responses in the event they occur. "Go through" them completely; the child must know they will no longer work. Try to have several strong contingencies available so the child will see that the session with you will be fun. If all falls apart, get out of the session by ending it on a good note, even if that "note" is several steps backwards. Then evaluate everything you did, the child did, and anything you believe may be important. Most critically, if you're not able to identify what went wrong, obtain assistance from the professional who modeled for you. Don't allow the unsuccessful situation to persist for any length of time. Incorrect practice will reestablish the strength of the child's avoidance responses and, perhaps, teach her some new ones. That you do not need.

13. *You have mentioned a couple of times about holding the child's head when feeding. Do you always use restraint with a child who refuses to let you place a spoon in her mouth?*

I mentioned gently holding the child's head. You certainly do not want to cause the child pain when preventing her head from turning away from a spoon. The only purpose for using any restraining method is to help the child understand that her avoidance responses (head turning, clenching lips closed, etc.) will not work. Thus, the only time restraining called for is when you are working through the avoidance responses. If you are using a reinforcement contingency to help a child eat, restraining that produces discomfort would be counterproductive. You want the child to realize that she will gain access to the reinforcer by eating. You also want her to know that the reinforcer will be withheld if food is not consumed. You would use gentle restraint to get food into her mouth in order to provide her with the reinforcer. If the child is experiencing hunger and not experiencing any discomfort from eating, the need for restraining should be brief.

14. *Do you use any special approach with infants?*

I like to find a quiet location (particularly important in a special care unit) that is isolated and free from distractions. Frequently, I place the baby in a sitting position in an infant seat (small car seat). Other times, I'll have a nurse hold the child. I then experiment with various auditory, visual, and tactile toys to see if the infant has a preference. This is the experimental phase, which I hope will afford me an idea of what might be reinforcing to the child, and which is done prior to any attempt at feeding. Even with the very young baby, I want to have a strong contingency available. With a nurse or attending physician close by, I will place just a few drops of the child's formula on the infant's tongue, usually by way of a Brecht feeder. I then watch what the child does with the liquid. I'm looking for the point at which the child succeeds and the point at which the behavior breaks down. (This part of the exploration process is the same regardless of age.) Once I can find the precise point of success, I will introduce the contingency. Usually, the reinforcer is looking into a mirror, touching a stuffed animal, listening to music, or hearing soft, endearing words. Frequently, being rocked gently is highly valued by the child, but I prefer not to incorporate rocking as the reinforcing component of a contingency. During exploration/acquisition, the child must be able to discriminate precisely what he has done in order to receive the reinforcer. With a mirror or stuffed animal, learning the relationship between the behavior and the reinforcer is easy: the child swallows, the mirror or stuffed animal is provided immediately for a few seconds. But being rocked in someone's arms is too general a reinforcer. Invariably, the child is going to be rocked even when swallowing has not occurred. Further, simply being held may be as valued as being rocked, and by definition, once the child is placed in someone's arms, he is held regardless of what behavior is manifested. Again, during exploration/acquisition, we want the learning to take place as quickly and as comfortably as possible. For that to occur, the relationship between behavior and feedback must be clearly distinguishable. To help the child learn the components of the contingency, I will use multiple, brief sessions where I provide food to the child, followed immediately by the reinforcer. I can provide immediate feedback more readily and accurately with toys, lights, and sounds. Rocking rarely allows the same precision.

Whether a nippled bottle will replace the Brecht feeder is up to the child. After a few successful swallows with the Brecht feeder, I will try the nippled bottle. If the child fails to suck, I won't force the issue. I'll either go back to the Brecht feeder, or with the physician's approval, I will try solids. Solids are often easier than liquids for the child to control, once the food is placed on his tongue. If the child will swallow the solids (a mixture of baby cereal and formula, with a pasty consistency thicker than yogurt), then I may use a sequence such as: a small amount of solids, followed by a few drops of formula, followed by a few moments of mirror time or playing with the stuffed animal. Gradually, I will try to help the youngster take a little more food (liquid and solid) before providing the reinforcer. However, process and success are absolutely essential, as is patience. (Throughout it all, the child receives lots of warm verbal strokes.)

If the child is being augmentatively fed along with the "po" program, the augmentative feeding always occurs after the "po" feeding period, and it never takes place in the precise location where the "po" efforts occurred. Also, if the child really loves the mirror or stuffed animal, harsh as it may appear, I request that the artificial reinforcer be provided to the child only during the "po" feeding period. Once the child's eating has come under the control of natural feedback, the child can live with the mirrors and toys as long as desired.

15. *Do you suggest anything special with the infant in intensive care who is only a few weeks old?*

Most important, don't just do nothing: don't place the child off in a figurative corner and wait inactively until he's been given the green light to start "po" feeding. Practice with as many parts of "po" feeding as the child can tolerate and learn from: stimulating the child's mouth and tongue, introducing a pacifier to elicit sucking when the child is being augmentatively fed, posturing and positioning associated with feeding, and any number of other "feeding-like" experiences that I hope will help the neonate understand part of what "po" feeding is about. Try to make the infant's environment pleasant, as free from negative stimuli as is feasible. Plan regular, consistent "feeding" times where a routine is introduced to the infant as though feeding will take place, where a bottle, bib, food smells, and the like are brought into the infant's awareness. Eventually, the child will be exposed to "po" feeding, and the above preparation may make the introduction easier.

16. *Do you do anything special with the older child, the one who leaves the dinner table when he wants to, comes back when he wants to, eats what he wants to, and generally makes dinner time less than pleasurable for everyone but himself?*

Yes, I don't let him do it. I wouldn't allow it to happen if he was 2 or 22. In my view, parents must develop certain expectations for their child's eating behavior, just as they have expectations for bedtime activities, homework activities, and the like. While there aren't any cookbooks that can (or should) tell parents what guidelines to follow or what rules to impose, there are many books, written by highly competent professionals, suggesting that some clearly stated guidelines that provide limits for children's behaviors need to be in place. The guidelines' specifics must be determined, preferably jointly, by the parents. Assuming I was the parent of the child you mentioned in the question, my wife and I would sit with him well before dinner and explain which behaviors would be acceptable and which ones would not be tolerated. I would describe the behaviors carefully. If necessary I would model for the child what I wanted. I would ask the child to tell me what he was expected to do and avoid doing. If necessary, I would have him show me what I wanted. Then I would explain the reinforcement contingencies I intended to use. My child would know how his mother and I intended to respond to both his desired and undesired behaviors. He would learn very quickly that it would be in his best interests to abide by the rules established by his parents.

17. *How about the older child who wishes to eat only sweets?*

The child is not allowed to eat only sweets. Nor is she allowed to eat only corn on the cob or only steak or only pizza. She may certainly have candy, cake, and ice cream (corn, steak, and pizza), but only in conjunction with other foods. But what if she objects to your guidelines? Then you have a compliance problem. You will need to evaluate your use of type-one and type-two requests, along with the reinforcement contingencies that are (or are not) being employed. The message is straightforward: parents need to establish, through good communication, rules and regulations governing the behavior of their children. The children need to know how they are expected to behave. As I see it, the sooner the parents begin communicating and implementing the carefully thought out rules and limits, the better for everyone.

18. *Is it true that at home you prefer the young child to be fed in a high chair rather than while being held in someone's arms?*

Yes. A high chair provides more structure to the feeding scenario, an essential addition during exploration/acquisition and the beginnings of maintenance. Further, it is often much easier for the primary feeder to effectively deal with the child's avoidance responses (twisting, pushing, flailing) when the child is placed securely and comfortably in a high chair. And one more reason: the high chair provides a little "distance" between the feeder and the child. I've seen a few held children get squeezed rather painfully when they have failed to do as the feeder desired. Sometimes, a little distance provides the frustrated adult with a chance to cool off. Adding pain to a feeding sequence is disastrous for all involved.

19. *I'm an occupational therapist working with several children: one won't suck, one eats only very selected foods, and one won't eat at all. Quick suggestions?*

Have all three undergo a thorough medical examination. Check for aspirating, refluxing, swallowing difficulties, chewing difficulties, colic, and anything else a physician suggests. Remember, all children are supposed to eat. It is a natural behavior. If it is not happening, something is wrong. If:

    a. All three receive a clean bill of health;
    b. You are assured that the children have empty stomachs;
    c. You understand that process learning is much more important than quantity of food initially consumed; and
    d. You want to try something "quick"; then:

For the child who won't suck: get rid of the nipple. Try delivering liquids with a syringe, Brecht feeder, or cup. Try solids. Find a contingency. Remember, if the child has been augmentatively fed, he may have no idea that "po" feeding reduces hunger. Teach him that through brief, multiple, successful "po" sessions.

With the picky eater: develop a reinforcement contract. He gets what he wants after he eats what you want. First, give him a *small* taste of his favorite food; then give him another; then, quickly, give him a small taste of "your" food, followed immediately by his favorite. Both go into the mouth almost simultaneously. Tell him how great he's doing. Give him his food, then yours, then his. "Go through" any avoidance behaviors. Gradually require that he take two small tastes of your food before he gets a sizable taste of his. Brief, multiple, successful sessions. (Don't try this approach with Brussels sprouts. It won't work, unless they are the reinforcers.)

For the noneater: find a very strong artificial reinforcer. Find the point at which the child succeeds on the eating sequence.

Wherever that point is, show him how to earn the reinforcer: "After the empty spoon touches your lips, you can play for a few seconds." Move up the sequence: "After the empty spoon touches your tongue, you can play for a few seconds." And so on. "This first," you tell the child, "then this." Stay with it. Work through the avoidance responses. Do not allow the child to have what he wants until after he has done what you want. But . . . don't ask the child to do something that he's not capable of doing. That will become a no-win situation for you both.

20. *I've often wondered whether these food-refusing children have any conception of when feeding is to start and when it is going to stop.*

Most, I would suspect, know when feeding is going to start: they see the food, the bib, the high chair, the spoon, and the like. When the session will stop? Probably a complete mystery. Further, it's not likely they have the foggiest notion of how much or how little they are expected to eat.

The kids need cues. Some consistent, predictable sign that helps them understand that feeding will not last for the remainder of their lives, that they are not expected to eat the contents of every opened jar in sight or every morsel of food placed on a plate.

21. *Some children seem to be very stubborn when it comes to feeding. Can a child's personality explain why she doesn't eat?*

Child development research clearly indicates that beginning in the womb, children do manifest observable personality differences. But suggesting that stubbornness or any similar quality or characteristic is responsible for an absence of eating is (1) highly problematic, (2) of little practical use and (3) an example of circular logic—Why doesn't the child eat? Because she's stubborn. How do you know she's stubborn? Because she doesn't eat. Oh.

In all likelihood, the "stubborn" child is testing out the contingencies being used. She's learned in the past how stubborn she has to be before the primary feeder changes his or her mind. While stubborn is an acceptable description, smart would do just as well.

If the youngster appears stubborn, watch what you're doing. Do you stick with your contingencies, or do you change them after growing tired of the child's food-refusing behavior? Are you working through the avoidance responses, or are you requiring that the child exercise them for a lengthy period before you, once again, grow tired and give in to the situation? By changing contingencies when the child fails to do what you want and by allowing the avoidance responses to win, you effectively teach the child to become more stubborn (read persistent).

22. *Does everyone use your approach with food-refusing children?*

I am sure that every professional who works directly with these children is attempting to do much of what I have advocated: make sure the child's not experiencing any pain from eating; increase hunger drive; and show the child how to gain access to both artificial and natural feedback that will help maintain "po" feeding. We are all trying to show the children that eating can be enjoyable, that it is not something to fear or avoid. We are all trying to bring the child's eating under control of the natural environment.

23. *Have you been able to identify your own methods and personality characteristics that you believe have helped you experience success with many of these food-refusing children?*

I've had an opportunity while working with many of the children to watch myself on videotape. I've also had a chance to watch numerous parents and professionals as they, too, have worked with the children. After looking and comparing, I think I've been able to identify several variables that I incorporate that may be potentially valuable. I have only anecdotal data to support my beliefs, however.

    a. My reactions are very quick. I respond to the child's behavior immediately. When I'm sitting across from the child, I'm "on."
    b. I rarely miss anything the child does. I watch her every

movement, every reaction; I work hard to find something positive about her actions. I pay particular attention to any approximations that she might manifest that I can build upon. If I find one, I get to it immediately. I am a "hyper" kind of person. I think that is somewhat of an advantage. I must be prepared to move quickly when seeing something important.

c. I'm very firm, very affectionate; I'm fun, but forthright. I block out everyone around me. I try to figuratively tie a cord between the child and myself: I want her to feel my energy; I want her to draw support from my confidence. I try to tell her through actions, words, and facial expressions, that, "We're in this together. You're going to eat. Let's make the exercise as enjoyable as possible."

d. I'm particularly sensitive to the development of contingencies. I'm constantly on the alert for one that will work for the child. Again, I watch the child's every move. Somewhere within all that is going on, the child will tell me what she values. If I learn that, and if I have discovered the level at which the child can succeed, the child and I are on our way.

e. I'm very patient, very optimistic.

f. I use lots of small sessions. I try to make each one exciting and fun (not always possible, of course). If the child has been a total food refuser, I might be very satisfied if she will let me touch a spoon to her lips. If she allows a drop of food to her tongue, that might be more than enough for the moment. I've ended a session after a child swallowed 3 or 4 spoonfuls of food, and I have judged that session to be successful. Sometimes I've ended a session after the child has just sat comfortably and looked (even smiled) at me for several minutes. I've shown her an important, beginning lesson: sitting in a chair with utensils and plates on the tray or table will not be accompanied by my screaming,

yelling, threatening, or anything frightening. For some
children, that is truly a successful experience.

g. I feel for the child. Most of them have gone through so
much. When I touch one of them, it's as though I'm
touching one of my own. I care for the child and perhaps the child senses that. At the same time, my deep
empathy for the child does not interfere with lessons I
want the youngster to learn or the approaches I intend
to use. A child's crying may pain me, but it will not
dissuade me from allowing it to run its course if ignoring it is in the best interests of the child. I may understand a child's acquired fear of a spoon or fork, but the
fear will not stop my efforts. To the contrary, that she
does fear those objects pushes me to help her relinquish those fears so she can go beyond them. The child
learns quickly that I am a friend. But the child also
learns that I expect certain things from her; that I will
not allow her previously experienced physical difficulties or presently described disabilities to weaken my
efforts or intentions. If anything, the difficulties become an impetus for me to push the child forward.
Friends do that. Friends do not allow the past to hold
back the present or future.

24. *I get the impression that ending a session on a positive note is truly
valuable.*

It is very important. I will go to nearly any means to get the
child to learn that he's done something "great" that has resulted in
the end of a session. If he's quiet for 10 seconds (after crying for 10
minutes, that's great), if he tastes a new food, swallows without
fussing, doesn't gag or try to smack me in the nose, that's all great.
I will get him out of the high chair in a wink. I'll get down on the
floor with him to play, sing, or dance. Again, I want him to know
that good things happen when he eats (or moves in that direction).
For some children, the good thing is just getting out of the high

chair. Ten seconds of quiet behavior will do it. As will any of the other "great" things just mentioned.

25. *Do you sometimes have to alter an approach because it is not working? Does the child become confused by the switching of approaches?*

I would say that it is extremely rare when I do *not* alter approaches. No more than a handful of the children were helped with their "po" feeding with the first method tried. Most required three or four adaptations before the "correct fit" was discovered. Regarding the issue of confusion? There may be some initial confusion when requirements or expectations are altered, but the kids are amazingly adaptive: assuming some ultimate consistency with an approach, the children seemed not to be bothered by the continual experimentation.

26. *How long should you stay with an approach before trying another?*

That is a very difficult question to answer. Sometimes you can tell instantly that you're on the wrong track. The child's behavior tells you: there's an increase in avoidance responses or a complete shut down in eating. The same child's behavior, however, can also tell you if you're on a better track. If he seems a drop more receptive, a drop less resistant, a drop happier, a drop less fussy, and he's eating or tasting or swallowing a drop or two more, you're probably doing what you should, and you probably should stick with it. It is very difficult to be more precise. Just remember, the bottom line is the child's behavior. Use the behavior to let you know how well you are doing. If things are going downhill, don't hesitate to brainstorm another approach.

27. *What do you do when nothing seems to work? What do you do when the child stops eating after she had begun to eat so well? What do you do when you think you've done everything?*

You take a break; you relax; you get away from feeding, food, bibs, forks, plates, and everything associated with them for an hour-long soak in the tub, a walk in a warm, green park, or 100 decibels of the Rolling Stones. Refreshed, smiling, you start once again from the very beginning. You ask yourself, and everyone involved, questions and more questions.

    a. How about natural feedback?
       1. Pleasant tastes?
       2. Reduction of hunger?
    b. Is the child hungry?
       1. Check calories?
       2. Check liquids?
    c. Any physical discomfort?
       1. Any yet-discovered physical problem?
    d. Any emotional discomfort?
    e. Process?
       1. Does the child understand what will happen when she eats?
       2. Does she know that swallowing reduces hunger?
    f. Incentives?
       1. Artificial reinforcers?
       2. Contingencies?
          a. Being used?
          b. Being used correctly?
    g. Avoidance responses?
       1. Who's winning?
    h. Am I asking too much too soon? Am I pushing too much too soon?
    i. Have I grown impatient?
    j. Can I find someone to watch what's happening?
    k. The child is telling me something. I'll find someone to help me figure out the message.

What do you do? You start again from step one. You get some help and you start again . . . from step one. The child will appreciate it.

Nutrition

Patty Reid, R.D.

Patty Reid is a registered dietitian at The Children's Hospital in Denver, Colorado. We have worked together on many of the cases described in this book. I have asked her to share information directly relating to food-refusal children, as well as offering her views on how to "punch up" foods and provide good nutrition for young children. She is married and is expecting her first child. In Patty's own words, "Nutritional assessment and management are essential components in the care of a food-refusing child. The registered dietitian works with the other members of an interdisciplinary team to provide optimal nutritional care. The beginning of this chapter will discuss the nutritional needs of the food refuser. In the second portion of the chapter, practical information used to develop the nutritional care plan will be highlighted."

Baseline Information

Nutritional History

The nutritional history is a tool for gathering information about a child's food consumption and eating behaviors. (The histo-

227

ry is most often secured during the initial interview.) Components of the nutritional history include information about diet from birth to the present, history of family and social situation, and a summary of the child's nutritional status.

Recall of Usual Food Intake

To obtain information about "usual" food intake, the parent might be asked by the dietitian, "Please tell me what your child usually eats and drinks on a typical day. Start with the first thing your child eats or drinks when he wakes in the morning." The child's food consumption throughout the day and night is then discussed. It is necessary to obtain estimates of food portions to enable evaluation of nutrient intake. Some practitioners prefer to obtain a 24-hour recall. This involves having the parent recall *all* food items consumed within the period of 24 hours. A major problem with food recalls is that they are retrospective, relying on the memory of the caregiver.[1]

Diet Record

A diet record is an ongoing, prospective record of a child's food intake that is usually kept for 3 days. The parents are asked to record the following information about their child's diet:

1. All food and fluids consumed.
2. Time of day food and liquids are consumed.
3. Method of food preparation (e.g., baking, frying).
4. Food portions (e.g., ounces, cups, teaspoons, tablespoons).

The diet record is often more accurate than the previous food recall method because food intake is recorded close to (or exactly at) the time of actual consumption. With paper and pencil, the parent writes down precisely what is consumed. Regardless of method used, once a food recall or diet record is obtained, the dietitian analyzes it for calorie, protein, and nutrient content. The assumption is made that if a child's intake appears adequate for growth, then growth can be expected. If growth does not occur despite satisfactory nutritional intake, the child should be examined thoroughly by the family physician to ascertain if organic problems are interfering with the child's progress.

A Point to Remember

A child may be consuming satisfactory quantities of food but he may not be receiving sufficient quality of food. Such is particularly possible when a child's total diet is composed of prepared formula. If an infant is being fed formula, it is critical to determine how the formula is being mixed. Parents should be given explicit, simple instructions regarding mixing formula that leave no room for confusion or ambiguity. Succinctly, improper formula preparation (or incorrectly diluted formula) can be the sole cause of insufficient weight gain in a child.

Nutritional Assessment

The following are some issues that directly relate to growth curves, ideal body weight, determination of preferred caloric and liquid intake, as well as other concerns often associated with the food-refusing child.

Body Measurements

Repeated body measurements over time provide important information regarding a child's personal growth. Such measurements allow the parent and physician to see how a child is prog-

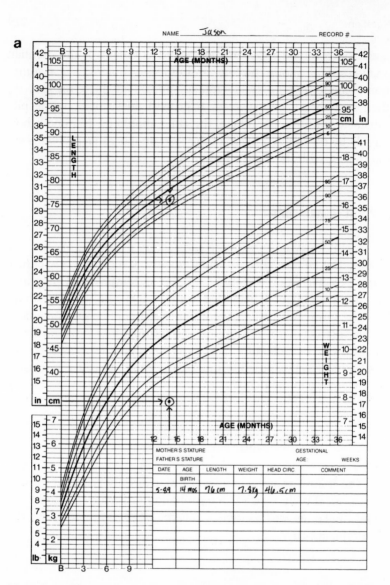

Figure 1. Physical growth National Center for Health Statistics (NCHS) percentiles based on weight and length for (a) boys, birth to 36 months and (b) girls, birth to 36 months. Adapted from Hamill *et al.*[2] Reprinted with permission of Ross Laboratories.

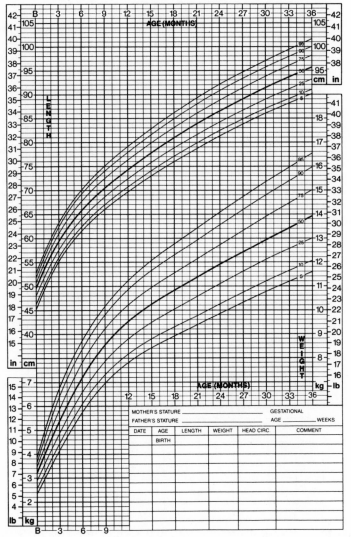

Figure 1. (*Continued*)

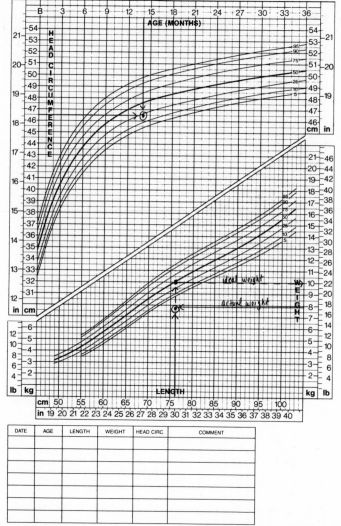

Figure 2. Physical growth National Center for Health Statistics (NCHS) percentiles based on head circumference and weight/length ratios for (a) boys, birth to 36 months and (b) girls, birth to 36 months. Adapted from Hamill *et al*.[2] Reprinted with permission of Ross Laboratories.

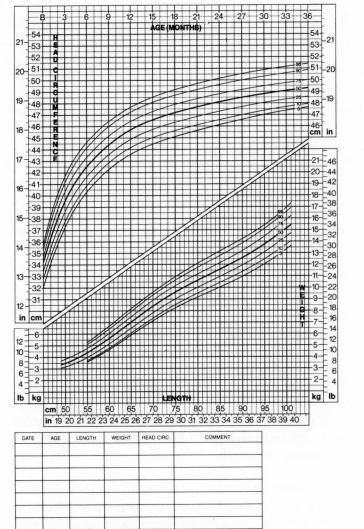

DATE	AGE	LENGTH	WEIGHT	HEAD CIRC.	COMMENT

Figure 2. *(Continued)*

ressing. The National Center for Health Statistics (NCHS) has established growth percentile curves based on large, nationally representative samples of children.[2] Growth charts, based on the NCHS standards, are used in evaluating a child's growth parameters. Figures 1a and 2a illustrate how length, weight, head circumference and weight-for-length ratios are plotted on the growth chart for our subject's age and sex. (Figures 1b and 2b represent charts to be used for female subjects.) If you would like to try plotting a weight-for-length ratio on a growth chart, see Figure 2a. Find the point where the lines extending from the child's weight (7.8 kilogram [kg]=17 lbs, 5 oz.) and length (76 centimeters [cm]=30 inches) intersect. (For your information, 1 kilogram equals 2.2 pounds, and 2.54 centimeters equals 1 inch.) This point of intersection is the child's weight-for-length ratio. In the example given, the weight-for-length ratio is less than the fifth percentile because it is under the line labeled "5." A weight-for-length ratio of less than the fifth percentile indicates that a child is underweight for height.

To determine a child's ideal body weight, find the line extending from the child's length. Locate the point where this line intersects the heavy line labeled "50." From this point, follow a horizontal line to the right until you reach the number indicating the child's ideal weight. The ideal body weight in the example given is 10 kg (22 pounds). As you might expect, determining parental and sibling height and weight provides information on a child's genetic predisposition for growth.

Interesting Points: (1) Children who are malnourished grow at a rate greater than expected for age when optimal nutrition is eventually provided. This phenomenon, called "catch-up growth," has been described throughout the literature.[3,4,5] The growth rate is rapid initially, then gradually declines until normal growth percentiles are achieved. (2) The goal for weight gain is 30 grams (1 ounce) per day in the infant and 60 to 90 grams (2 to 3 ounces) per day in the young child.[6]

Table 1. RDAs for Energy and Protein[a]

Please check with your child's pediatrician
to determine variations that might be best
for your child.

Age (years)	Energy needs (calories/kg)	Protein needs (grams/kg)
0.0–0.5	115	2.2
0.5–1.0	105	2.0
1–3	100	1.8
4–6	85	1.5
7–10	86	1.2

[a]*Source*: Adapted from National Research Council, Food
and Nutrition Board. *Recommended Dietary Allowances*,
9th edition. Washington, D.C.: National Academy of
Sciences, 1980.

Establishing Nutritional Goals

The Recommended Dietary Allowances (RDAs) are used as
the basis for calculating calorie needs per age group (see Table 1).
Two methods for establishing calorie needs are outlined. Either
method provides an acceptable estimate of calorie needs for catch-
up growth, which, research suggests, may be 50% greater than for
children who have maintained satisfactory weight growth.[7] To
help you understand how to determine caloric needs, sample
calculations will be shown using the body measurements of a 14-
month-old boy. His case will be described shortly. First, check
Table 1 again. Notice the caloric needs by age per measured weight
as reported in kilograms. (A child who is between one-half and a
full year of age will need roughly 105 calories for each kg of
weight.) Our 14-month-old boy has, as every child does, an "ideal"
body weight. If you will look at Figure 2a, you will see how this
child's ideal body weight was determined. You might wish to re-
read the explanation regarding the weight-for-length ratio described a little earlier. That, too, will help you determine an ideal
body weight.

Calorie needs, of course, are calculated on the basis of the ideal body weight measure. There is a formula that helps with this determination. The formula looks like this[8]:

Ideal body weight (kg) × RDA calories per kg for age =
total calorie needs per day.

In the case of the 14-month-old, his ideal body weight, given his length, is 10 kg. To figure his total calorie needs, simply locate his age (14 months) on Table 1 to determine the number of needed calories per kg. In his case the number is 100. The completed formula would look like this:

10 kg × 100 calories per kg = 1,000 calories per day

As indicated earlier there is a second method for determining needed calories per day that is used predominantly for catch-up growth. Notice that this formula carries a correction component of 1.5. This correction component, as may be obvious, will produce a higher calorie need per day. The formula looks like this:

Actual weight (kg) × RDA calories/kg for age × 1.5 =
total calories needed per day

Given our 14-month-old youngster (remember Table 1), and using his actual weight of 7.8 kilograms, the formula would look like this:

7.8 kg × 100 calories/kg × 1.5 = 1,170 calories per day

You can average the difference in the two results to determine caloric needs:

1000 + 1170 = 2,170 ÷ by 2 = 1,085

or you can select either figure, depending upon your preference or that of the child's physician. (You should always check with your physician for guidance and advice regarding your child's caloric/ nutritional needs.)

The RDAs are also used to calculate protein needs. Again using our 14-month-old, and checking Table 1, we can determine his total protein needs in grams (gm) per day. The formula looks like this:

Ideal body weight (kg) × protein (gm)/kg for age =
total protein in gm per day

Or with numbers:

10 kg × 1.8 gm/kg = 18 gm/day

Fluids

All this talk about proteins and calories may make you forget liquids. But it is essential to consider the fluid needs of a child when developing the nutritional care plan. The equation below is useful for calculating normal daily fluid requirements. (Again, a little practice will make it workable.) The formula, however, is not appropriate for conditions in which there are increased or decreased fluid needs or losses.[9] For example, fluid needs are increased during periods of diarrhea or hot weather. If you have particular questions about a child's fluid needs, check with the youngster's family physician or dietitian. The equation:

   100 cc*/kg for the first 10 kg of body weight,
plus   50 cc/kg for each kg of body weight from 10 to 20 kg,
       20 cc/kg for each additional kg over 20 kg of body weight.

*There are 30 ccs per 1 ounce.

Our 14-month-old:

7.8 kg × 100 cc/kg = 780 cc of fluid, which equals 26 ounces/day

Explanation: The 14-month-old weighs 7.8 kg. The equation says 100 ccs for the first 10 kg. Therefore, 7.8 kg × 100. Since the child does not weigh more than 10 kg, the calculation is complete. Simply multiply 7.8 times 100, which equals 780 ccs. If you'd like, divide 780 by 30, which equals 26 (30 ccs per ounce), and you end up with the number of fluid ounces needed per day.

Nutritional Intervention

An individual nutritional care plan is developed based on information gathered from the nutrition history, medical records, and feeding observations. The feeding plan must be carefully tailored to meet the needs of the individual child. In the short term, it will work better to enhance present eating habits and food preferences rather than trying to change them. For example, instead of trying to wean a child whose weight is poor off the bottle, try adding a higher-calorie beverage to the bottle to help promote weight gain. Once the child is gaining weight and succeeding with the present feeding plan, weaning from the bottle could then be attempted.

Snacks and Handouts

Frequent, brief feedings are appropriate for the infant and young child because their stomachs are small and their energy needs are high. A newborn infant will usually eat every 2 to 3 hours. A typical feeding routine for the toddler is: breakfast, mid-morning snack, lunch, afternoon snack, dinner, and bedtime snack. Note that a distinction has been made between what we call "planned snacks" and "handouts."[10] Having planned meals and snacks often teaches the child to expect the regular feedings as part of the daily routine. If a child is given frequent handouts, somewhat randomly, the youngster may not learn to eat what is served at meal time. Instead, the child will expect a snack shortly after an unfinished meal. Such an expectation can lead to all sorts of difficulties, many of which were discussed during earlier chapters. There's another point with random handouts also discussed earlier. A child who eats constantly because food is "there," may never fully experience a sensation of hunger because his stomach has something in it all the time. If a food-refusal problem presents itself at a later point in time, this potential absence of sensation can create difficulties unnecessarily. Additionally, time of meals and snacks should be consistent (although not completely rigid) from day to day, night to night. If there is a long span between meals, the child many need two snacks instead of one.

Interesting Points: (1) It is beneficial to allow about 1 hour without food or drink (except water) before a feeding to help stimulate the appetite. (2) Allowing 5 to 15 minutes of quiet time before a meal can help a child to settle down before the feeding. (3) An appropriate amount of time for a feeding is 20 to 30 minutes, unless, as indicated earlier, a shorter time facilitates acquisition of eating.

Fluid Consumption

Consumption of fluids in excess of calculated needs can lead to poor intake of solid food. If overconsumption of fluids is a problem, it may help to offer solids first at a feeding, followed by fluids. Beverages with empty calories (such as carbonated and sweetened beverages) are not recommended because they fill a child up and contribute few nutrients to the diet. A general rule of thumb is to limit fruit juice to 4 to 8 ounces per day in the diet of all food-refusing children who would drink juice rather than most anything else. Whole milk is encouraged to boost intake of calories and protein. It is acceptable to offer a child plain water for thirst, keeping fluid intake at a reasonable level.

Mealtime Environment

Creating a pleasant mealtime environment will increase the likelihood that feeding will become a positive experience for the child. It is ideal to put the young child in a high chair for all feedings and to limit distractions in the room (e.g., TV). Parents should not be afraid to allow their child to make a mess at feedings. Mess-making, when accomplished with fingers that go into the mouth, can promote self-feeding skills.

Vitamins and Minerals

The need for vitamin and mineral supplementation is evaluated on an individual basis. The child's diet is evaluated for nutritional adequacy and recommendations for supplementation are made. When possible, changes in the diet are made in order to obtain nutrients from the diet instead of from vitamin and mineral supplements. In some situations, it may be very reassuring for the parent to give the child a daily vitamin and mineral supplement, providing the supplement may help reduce parental anxiety regarding the child's poor eating habits. Parents should check with the child's physician before giving any supplement.

Nutrition Suggestions for Infants

Concentrating infant formulas above 20 calories per ounce is a way to boost the caloric content of an infant's diet. (The child's physician should also be consulted to determine if a special formula is necessary.) Formulas can be safely concentrated to 24 calories per ounce by adding less water to concentrated liquid or powdered formula. Formula with 24 calories per ounce can be prepared in either of the following ways: (1) take one can (13 ounces) of concentrated liquid formula and add 8 1/2 ounces of water, or (2) take 5 ounces of water and add three scoops of formula powder. Formulas should be concentrated to 27 or 30 calories per ounce only when the 24-calorie per ounce formula fails to provide enough calories for adequate growth and the formula volume cannot be increased.[11] Concentrating formulas from 24 to 30 calories per ounce should be accomplished by the inclusion of carbohydrate and/or fat within the formula. It is important to note that the 30-calorie per ounce formula (prepared by the method outlined above) is marginal in protein adequacy.[11] Less free water is available when formulas are concentrated; therefore, adequate fluid intake is essential. Parents need careful instructions regarding the preparation of concentrated formula. A child on a concentrated infant formula requires the supervision of a physician and/or dietitian.

Table 2 illustrates feeding guidelines for the infant's first year of life. The table shows how the infant's diet is progressed from formula or breast milk for the first 4 to 6 months of life to baby foods and gradually to table and finger foods. The table is a general guide that is meant to be tailored to the individual infant's needs. It is important for the parent and dietitian to use the information obtained from the nutritional history to plan a high-calorie diet for the infant. The foods accepted by one 9-month-old child can be quite different from those accepted by another same-aged child.

Commercial Baby Foods and Diets

Commercial baby foods vary in their caloric content. It is very useful for parents to read the labels of baby foods and choose the items that are higher in calories. For example, a 4.5-ounce jar of

Table 2. Food for Baby's First Year[a]

The foods that a baby can eat depends on the baby's developmental readiness and nutritional needs. This table is intended to serve as a guide. It is important to confer with your pediatrician to determine precisely what foods your baby needs.

Birth (the baby suckles)	Breast milk; iron-fortified infant formula

4–6 months
   (baby controls head
   movement)
	Iron fortified infant cereal

5–7 months (sits with support)	Strained or pureed fruits and vegetables

6–8 months
   (sits with support)
	Strained or pureed meat, chicken, fish, beans,
	   cottage cheese, plain yogurt, cooked egg yolk,
	   tofu

7 months (chews)	Diluted fruit juice from a cup

7–9 months
   (grasps and holds)
	Other infant cereals (wheat/mixed grains),
	   mashed fruits and vegetables, finger foods:
	   toast squares, unsalted soda crackers, soft tor-
	   tilla, cooked vegetable strips or slices, peeled,
	   soft fruit wedges or slices, cheese cubes

9–12 months (improves coordination)	Mashed or chopped food from the family meal
1 year (feeds self)	Introduce whole milk and whole egg. (Offer 3 meals a day plus a snack.)

[a]Source: Adapted from Colorado Department of Health Nutrition Services. Reprinted with permission.

strained sweet potatoes contains 80 calories per jar, whereas a 4.5-ounce jar of strained carrots contains 40 calories per jar. Every bite of sweet potatoes a child eats will have twice as many calories as each bite of carrots. A 4.5-ounce jar of strained bananas with tapioca contains 110 calories per jar versus 60 calories per jar for strained applesauce. In general, plain, strained meats or blended homemade meats have more calories than strained vegetable-meat combinations. One ounce of commercial strained chicken contains 44 calories, whereas 1 ounce of strained chicken-vegetable dinner contains only 18 calories. Baby food desserts (ranging from 90 to 120 calories per 4.5-ounce jar) are acceptable in moderation. Obviously, if a child's diet is solely composed of desserts, it will be lacking in nutrients. Homemade baby foods should also be selected for high calorie content. A parent can obtain information on calorie content of homemade baby food from a dietitian.

"Punch-Up" Foods

"Punch-up" foods can be added to an infant's diet to boost calories. They need to be age and/or developmentally appropriate; therefore, the "punch-up" foods recommended for infants are more limited than those suggested in Table 3 for children over 1 year of age. This is because an infant's digestive system and oral motor skills may not be mature enough to handle many of the foods shown in Table 3.

Adding fats (butter, margarine, or oil) to an infant's food will add approximately 40 calories per teaspoon. (Check with your physician to see if adding fats is contraindicated, given your youngster.) The 4.5-ounce jar of sweet potatoes that contains 80 calories per jar will provide 120 calories per jar if one teaspoon of butter or margarine is melted and mixed in. By adding the teaspoon of fat, the caloric density of the sweet potatoes has increased by 50% without increasing the volume of the food. Formula powder (44 calories per scoop) can be added to table foods such as yogurt or mashed potatoes. Adding one scoop of formula powder to 2 ounces of fruited yogurt increases the calories from 64 to 108. Adding once scoop of formula powder to 1/4 cup of mashed potatoes boosts calories from 40 to 84 per serving. Infant cereals and dehydrated infant foods can be prepared with formula instead of water to increase calories. Four tablespoons of baby rice cereal mixed with 2 ounces of water equals 60 calories. The same amount of cereal mixed with infant formula and topped with 1 teaspoon of butter or margarine has 140 calories per serving. One serving (3

Table 3. "Punch-Up" Foods[a]

Food	Calories/tablespoon
Fats	
Oil	120
Butter	108
Margarine	102
Mayonnaise	99
Peanut butter	86
Heavy whipping cream	52
Cream cheese	50
Cheese spread	47
Sour cream	26
Half & half cream	20
Milk	
Sweetened condensed	62
Evaporated, undiluted	21
Powdered skim	16
Sweets	
Honey	61
Corn syrup	57
Jam and jelly	55
Brown sugar	52
Maple syrup	50
White sugar	48

[a]*Source*: Pennington, J. A., & Church, H. N. (1985). *Food values of portions commonly used*. Philadelphia: Lippincott.

tablespoons) of dehydrated banana flakes reconstituted with equal parts of water has 50 calories. Mixing the banana flakes with formula instead of water provides 80 calories. By carefully planning the infant's diet, total calories in the diet can be increased without increasing the volume of food an infant needs to eat. This concentration of calories will help promote the desired catch-up growth.

Nutrition Suggestions for Children over 1 Year of Age

An example of a daily guide for feeding children age one and over is shown in Tables 4 and 5. A child's diet over time is more

Table 4. Foodchart: An Example of a Child-Care Food Program[a]

The following represent minimal quantities. Check with your child's pediatrician to determine if the suggested quantities and types are suited for your child.

	Amount per age group		
Foods	1–3 yrs	3–6 yrs	6–12 yrs
Breakfast			
Fluid milk	½ cup	¾ cup	1 cup
Juice *or* fruit *or* vegetable	¼ cup	½ cup	½ cup
Bread *or* bread alternate	½ slice	½ slice	1 slice
Snack (serve 2)			
Fluid milk	½ cup	½ cup	1 cup
Juice[b] *or* fruit *or* vegetable	½ cup	½ cup	¾ cup
Meat *or* meat alternate	½ ounce	½ ounce	1 ounce
Bread *or* bread alternate	½ slice	½ slice	1 slice
Lunch/dinner			
Fluid milk	½ cup	¾ cup	1 cup
Meat *or* poultry *or* fish *or*	1 ounce	1 ounce	1 ounce
Cheese *or*	1 ounce	1½ ounce	2 ounces
Egg *or*	1	1	1
Cooked dry beans and peas *or*	¼ cup	⅜ cup	½ cup
Peanut butter	2 tbsp	3 tbsp	4 tbsp
Vegetables and/or fruits[c]	¼ cup	½ cup	¾ cup
Bread *or* bread alternate	½ slice	½ slice	1 slice

[a]*Source*: Colorado Department of Health-CCFP, 1987. Reprinted with permission.
[b]Juice may not be served if milk is the only other component at snack.
[c]Must serve at least two different varieties and a minimum of ⅛-cup each must be served.

important than what is eaten on an individual day. A child who does not consume the minimal number of servings from each food group on one day will probably make up for it in the next day or two—one reason for not requiring a child to finish everything on her plate during a particular meal. (Such variability is not a problem unless a strong aversion to one food group develops. If so, it is best to deal with the food refusal before it creates any concerns.) It is important to note that serving sizes listed are child-size portions, not adult portions. It is much better if a child finishes her meal and asks for seconds rather than being given portions so large she

Table 5. A Guide for Feeding the 1- to 5-year-old[a]

Foods appropriate for any child will vary depending upon the child's developmental level and nutritional needs. Be certain to check with your child's pediatrician to determine which foods are best for your child.

Breakfast:
   Fruit or juice (preferably high in vitamin C)
   Egg or cereal with milk
   Bread, toast, or tortilla
   Milk
Noon meal:
   Protein food
   Raw or cooked vegetable
   Bread or tortilla
   Milk
   Fruit
Evening meal:
   Protein food
   Vegetables: 1 raw, 1 cooked
   Bread or tortilla
   Milk
What makes a good snack?
   1. Food from one or more of the food groups, such as: fruit, raw vegetables, crackers, fruit juice, peanut butter, cheese, nuts.
   2. Foods that are low in sugar.
   3. Small amounts of food that don't spoil the appetite for meals.

[a]The following foods are not recommended for children under age 3 because they may cause choking: raw vegetables, grapes, nuts, seeds, popcorn, raisins, hot dogs, tough meat, berries, hard candy. *Source*: Adapted from Colorado Department of Health Nutrition Services. Reprinted with permission.

cannot finish them and feels frustrated. It is important to introduce new foods in very small portions.

Foods from the milk group are a good source of protein, riboflavin, and calcium. If a child is not a milk lover, foods such as cheese, flavored milk, and yogurt are good substitutes. Custard, pudding, and ice cream are high-calorie food choices from the milk group. Meat contributes protein, iron, and B vitamins to the diet. Children do not require large portions of meat to satisfy their protein needs. If a child is drinking 2 cups of milk per day, a toddler can meet his protein needs with 1 ounce of meat per day, a preschooler with 2 ounces, and a school-aged child with 3 ounces per day.[11] Fruits and vegetables add vitamins A and C and fiber to the diet. Children frequently like fruits better than vegetables. Rather than fighting about vegetable consumption, offer the child a small amount of vegetables at meals along with another good source of vitamin A, such as peaches or cantaloupe. Remember to avoid filling a child up with too much fruit juice. A child who recently has consumed 6 ounces of juice may not be particularly hungry for lunch or dinner. Breads and grains, rich in B vitamins and iron, are generally well accepted by the young child. It is good to include some whole grain bread and cereals in the child's diet, but do not go overboard with fiber. High-fiber diets, frequently recommended for adults, are not appropriate for young children. Excessive amounts of fiber in the diet can interfere with nutrient absorption, fill up a child too quickly, and cause gas or diarrhea. Foods high in fiber (fruits, vegetables, and grains) are generally low in calories.

It is important to select a high-calorie beverage as part of the food-refuser's diet. There is nothing wrong with keeping a child on a concentrated infant formula past the age of 1 year. If a child is milk intolerant, the soy-based infant formula should be continued past 1 year of age as a good source of calories and nutrients. For the child drinking milk, whole milk should be provided. "Double-strength" milk can be prepared by mixing 8 ounces of whole milk with 2 tablespoons of powdered milk, increasing to 4 tablespoons of powdered milk as tolerated. Signs of intolerance to a formula include vomiting, abdominal distention, or diarrhea.

Instant breakfast powder can also be added to whole milk, starting with 1/2 package instant breakfast per 8 ounces of whole milk, increasing to 1 package as tolerated. Ross Laboratories manufactures PediaSure, a nutritional supplement designed for the 1- to 6-year-old child. There are many, many adult nutritional supplements on the market. It is essential to seek the advice of a dietitian or physician to determine which product is most suitable for the individual child. If a nutritional supplement is the child's sole source of nutrition, it must be carefully evaluated for nutritional adequacy. Adult products often do not meet the nutrient needs of children.

Practical "Punch Ups"

Table 3 lists punch-up foods which can be added to other foods to increase their caloric density. Table 6 shows examples of high-calorie finger foods, solids, and beverages. Frequently a child is unable to consume large quantities of food; therefore, concentration of calories is a useful technique.

1. Mix 8 ounces of fruit-flavored yogurt with 4 ounces of whole milk to make a yogurt smoothie.
2. Add marshmallows and whipping cream to hot chocolate.
3. "Super" pudding can be prepared by mixing 1 box instant pudding (3 3/4-ounce box), 2 cups of whole milk, 1/2 cup powdered milk, and 2 tablespoons of oil. Mix well and chill.
4. Canned eggnog is available year round.
5. Cheese cake with fruit topping is a tasty snack or dessert.
6. Offer chocolate milk if your child refuses plain whole milk. It has all the nutrition and extra calories.
7. Be creative with milkshakes. Start with ice cream and add whole milk or cream, powdered milk or instant breakfast powder, a small amount of oil, fruit flavorings, etc.
8. Add (or melt) cheese on to everything you can think of—sandwiches, crackers, hamburgers, eggs, casseroles, vegetables, and sauces.
9. Deviled eggs make a fun finger food for snack time.
10. Add powdered milk to hot cereal, pancake mix, casseroles, mashed potatoes, baked goods, and meat patties.

Table 6. Calorie Content of Selected Foods[a]

Food	Amount	Calories
Dairy		
Eggnog	4 oz	171
Super pudding	¼ cup	140
Whole milk with instant breakfast	4 oz	140
Hot chocolate with 1 marshmallow	4 oz	134
Cheese cake	½ slice	128
Fruit-flavored yogurt	4 oz	127
Yogurt smoothie	4 oz	110
Double strength whole milk	4 oz	107
Whole chocolate milk	4 oz	104
Pudding made with whole milk	¼ cup	89
Custard	¼ cup	77
Whole milk	4 oz	75
Ice cream	¼ cup	74
Cheddar cheese	½ oz	57
Protein		
Pizza	1 slice	185
Deviled egg	1 egg	112
Sausage	1 oz	109
Pork chop	1 oz	105
Bologna	1 slice	94
Tuna salad (oil packed)	¼ cup	92
Hamburger patty	1 oz	78
Chicken drumstick	1 oz	65
Fish stick	1 oz	58
Fruits/vegetables		
Apple with 1 tablespoon of peanut butter	¼ apple	106
Corn with 1 teaspoon of margarine	¼ cup	78
Avocado	¼ med	77
Peach in 1 tablespoon of heavy cream	¼ peach	61
Raisins	2 tbsp	57
Broccoli with 1 tablespoon of cheese sauce	¼ cup	54
Banana	½ med	53

(continued)

Table 6. (*Continued*)

Food	Amount	Calories
Carrots in 1 teaspoon of butter sauce	¼ cup	47
Grains		
Blueberry muffin with 1 teaspoon of butter	½ muf	97
Graham cracker with 1 tablespoon cream cheese	1	80
Saltines with 1 tablespoon of cheese spread	2	73
Cream of Wheat with 1 teaspoon of butter	¼ cup	69
Oatmeal cookie	½	40

ᵃSource: Pennington, J. A., & Church, H. N. (1985). *Food values of portions commonly used.* Philadelphia: Lippincott.

11. Try cutting luncheon meats into shapes with cookie cutters.
12. Put a scoop of cottage cheese, egg salad, or tuna salad in an ice-cream cone.
13. Don't think of pizza as junk food. It is a good source of calories and protein . . . and lots of kids love it.
14. Ripe avocado slices are high-calorie finger foods that most parents do not think of providing.
15. Raisins can be eaten alone or added to other foods to boost calories and iron.
16. How about creamy peanut butter on apple slices or banana?
17. Serve peaches, strawberries, or other fruit in heavy cream.
18. Serve cooked vegetables with something on them, such as butter, margarine, sour cream, cheese sauce, or cream sauce.
19. Cook hot cereal with cream instead of water. Top the

cereal with a pat of butter or margarine and a sprinkle of sugar.

20. Never offer a plain cracker or piece of bread. Top them with something—cheese spread, cream cheese, butter, margarine, peanut butter, jelly, or honey.

21. Use real mayonnaise instead of salad dressing, because it has almost twice the calories.

22. Add butter or margarine to rice, pasta, Spaghetti-O's, and mashed potatoes.

23. Add a large dollop of whipping cream to Jello, pudding, fruits, and other desserts.

24. Bake cookies with nutritious ingredients such as oatmeal, raisins, and wheat germ.

25. Use cream or evaporated milk when preparing custards, puddings, or cream soups.

A Word of Caution: Choking is the fourth leading cause of accidental death in children under the age of 5 years in the United States. Slippery, round, often hard foods, peanuts, and small, hard candies, for example, are difficult for young children to hold in their mouths and chew, and they could lodge in the esophagus. When serving foods such as raisins, peanut butter, and apple slices to young children, adult supervision is recommended.

When high-fat punch-up foods are discussed with parents, a common reaction is, "Aren't these foods going to promote early heart disease?" Fats are a concentrated source of calories, containing 2 1/2 times more calories for a given amount than either carbohydrate or protein. The addition of fats to boost calories is a short-term technique used to treat the immediate problem of insufficient calories in the diet. Once a food-refusing child's eating behaviors are improved, the use of high-fat foods can be decreased to a moderate level. Neither the American Academy of Pediatrics[12] nor the American Heart Association[13] recommends a fat restricted diet for children under the age of 2.

Case Study: Jason

Keep in mind that the following case is only one example of nutrition intervention. It is intended to serve as a model. It is important for the parent and dietitian to design a nutrition care plan for each individual child to avoid deficiencies or excesses of nutrients.

Nutrition and Medical History

Jason is a 14-month-old male who was referred to The Children's Hospital outpatient clinic for evaluation of poor growth. Review of the medical records indicated that Jason was basically a healthy child with the exception of minor ear infections at 10 and 12 months of age.

The child's nutritional history from birth to the present was discussed with the youngster's parents. Jason was on iron-fortified infant formula from birth to 1 year of age. At 1 year, he was begun on whole milk. Solids were introduced at 6 months of age. According to the parents, Jason was never very eager to eat solids; instead, he always preferred to drink from his bottle. At present, he takes occasional sips from a cup during mealtimes. The parents report that their son has no problem with diarrhea, constipation, vomiting, chewing, or swallowing. He has no known food allergies and receives a vitamin and mineral drop each day. He is not on any medications and has not been hospitalized since his birth. He lives at home with his parents, has no siblings, and goes to day care 2 days per week for 7 hours per day. Medical exams have failed to find any physiological contraindications to normal "po" feeding and weight gain.

The provided recall of usual food intake representing a typical day indicated the following:

7:00 a.m.	8 ounces of whole milk
8:00 a.m. (breakfast)	1/4 slice plain toast; 15 Cheerios with 1 tablespoon of whole milk

10:00 a.m.	8 ounces of apple juice
12:00 p.m. (lunch)	1/4 cup of applesauce
2:00 p.m.	8 ounces of whole milk
5:00 p.m. (dinner)	2–3 bites of chicken or other meats; 2–3 bites of vegetables; 1/4 cup of ice cream
8:00 p.m.	4 ounces of whole milk

The above provides: 750 calories, 29 grams of protein, 840 ccs (28 ounces) of fluids

Nutritional Assessment

Jason's body measurements, plotted in Figures 1a and 2a, were as follows:

Length: 76 cm (30 inches)—25th percentile
Weight: 7.8 kg (17 lbs, 5 oz)—less than 5th percentile
Head circumference: 46.5 cm (18-1/3 inches)—25th percentile
Weight-for-length ratio: less than 5th percentile
Ideal body weight: 10 kg (22 lbs)

Parents' body measurements:

Mother's height: 165 cm (65 inches); weight: 61.4 kg (135 lbs)
Father's height: 178 cm (70 inches); weight: 70.5 kg (155 lbs)

Observation of a feeding session revealed that Jason had no problems chewing or swallowing. He demonstrated appropriate feeding skills. It became apparent that Jason was a partial food-refusing child. He would feed himself a few bites of food, but he would push away the spoon when his parents would attempt feeding. He would indicate his interest in his bottle. His parents often provided it without insisting that solids also be consumed.

Nutritional Goals

Calculations of Jason's calorie, protein, and fluid needs were as follows:

1. Calories: 1,000 to 1,170 per day
2. Protein: 18 grams per day
3. Fluids: 780 ccs (26 ounces) per day
4. Weight gain: approximately 0.5 kg (1.1 lbs) per week

From the recall of food intake, it was assessed that Jason was consuming adequate fluids and protein, but insufficient calories.

Nutritional Intervention

A consult was established with the hospital's "feeding team" to discuss behavioral intervention. The instituted plan was effective in increasing the child's willingness to consume more calories through solid foods. The dietitian then met with Jason's parents to provide a nutrition care plan.

1. Provide three meals and three snacks per day. Omit 7:00 a.m. bottle before breakfast.
2. Offer solids before liquids at mealtimes. Continue with "this first" contingencies developed by team.
3. Provide 22 ounces of whole milk per day. (Double strength whole milk or instant breakfast was not included because Jason's protein intake was already greater than adequate.)
4. Limit fruit juice to 8 ounces per day.
5. Aim for a variety of foods from all four food groups.
6. Fortify the foods Jason presently enjoys with punch-up foods.
7. Do not try to wean Jason from the bottle at the present time. Use it less often throughout each meal as solid food intake is increased.
8. Continue the daily vitamin and mineral supplement.

The dietitian and Jason's parents thoroughly discussed the nutrition care plan. Together they planned the following menu that would serve as model for home use.

8:00 a.m. (breakfast) 1/2 slice of toast with 1 teaspoon of margarine; 1/4 cup Cream of Wheat with 2 ounces of half-and-half and 1 teaspoon of sugar; 4 ounces of whole milk.

10:00 a.m. 4 ounces of orange juice; 1 graham cracker square with 1 tablespoon cream cheese.

12:00 p.m. (lunch) 1/4 tuna salad sandwich with mayonnaise; 1/2 banana; 4 ounces of whole milk.

2:00 p.m. 4 ounces of whole milk; 1/4 sliced soft peach with 1 tablespoon of heavy cream.

5:00 p.m. (dinner) 1/2 ounce of beef with 1 tablespoon of gravy; 2 tablespoons of potato with 1 tablespoon of gravy; 2 tablespoons of corn with 1/2 teaspoon of margarine; 4 ounces of whole milk.

8:00 p.m. 6 ounces of whole milk; 1/2 oatmeal cookie.

The above provides: 1,150 calories, 36 grams of protein, and 840 ccs (28 ounces) of fluid.

The dietitian, Jason, and his parents scheduled weekly follow-up sessions to monitor progress and weight gain and to make adjustments in foods if necessary. The program proved to be successful. Jason's food refusal decreased significantly, and his body weight improved steadily.

References

1. Mason, M., Wenberg, B. G, and Welsch, R. K. (1977). *The dynamics of clinical dietetics.* New York: John Wiley & Sons.
2. Hamill, P.V., Drizd, T. A., Johnson, C. L., Reed, R. B., Roche, A. F., and Moore, W. M. (1979). Physical growth: National Center For Health Statistics percentiles. *American Journal of Clinical Nutrition, 32,* 607–629.
3. Pipes, P. L. (1985). *Nutrition in infancy and childhood.* St. Louis: Times Mirror/Mosby College Publishing.
4. Peterson, K. E., Washington, J., and Rathbun, J. M. (1984). Team management of failure to thrive. *Journal of the American Dietetic Association, 84,* 810–815.
5. Goldbloom, R. B. (1982). Failure to thrive. *Pediatric Clinics of North America, 29,* 151–166.
6. Murray, C. A., and Glassman, M. S. (1982). Nutrient requirements during growth and recovery from failure to thrive. In P. J. Arcardo (ed.), *Failure to thrive in infancy and early childhood.* Baltimore: University Park Press.

7. Whitehead, R. G. (1977). Protein and energy requirements of young children in developing countries to allow catch-up growth after infection. *American Journal of Clinical Nutrition, 30*, 1545–1547.

8. Hohenbrink, K., and Oddleifson, N. (1989). Pediatric nutrition support. In E. D. Shronts (ed.), *Nutrition support dietetics.* Silver Spring: American Society for Parenteral and Enteral Nutrition.

9. Johns Hopkins Hospital, P.C. Rowe (ed.) (1987). *The Harriet Lane handbook.* Chicago: Year Book Medical Publishers.

10. Satter, E. (1987). *How to get your kid to eat . . . but not too much.* Palo Alto: Bull Publishing.

11. Breedon, C. (1986). Increasing the caloric density of infant formula. *Nutrition News, 1*, 1–6.

12. American Academy of Pediatrics, Committee On Nutrition (1986). Prudent lifestyle for children: Dietary fat and cholesterol. *Pediatrics, 78*, 521–525.

13. American Heart Association. (1983). Diet in the healthy child. *Circulation, 67*, 1411A–1414A.

CHAPTER TEN

Cases

The following cases are intended to provide further examples of problems and potential solutions to feeding difficulties seen with the food-refusal child. The cases are presented because of one or more unique aspects that may ring of circumstances similar to some you are facing. Additionally, the cases enable me to present a few ideas not previously covered.

COREY

Note how important it is for parents to make decisions about whether they are satisfied with how their child eats specifically and behaves in general. Problems with behavior, particularly for the older child, can present hardships for the entire family. Often, parents eventually choose to intervene in behalf of their food-refusal child for reasons other than weight gain and nutrition.

The 5-year-old was not thrilled to meet with me. "Do you know why you are here?" I asked him as we both sat on the floor of my office.

"Talk about food," he answered quietly. His mother, seated close by, smiled.

"What are we going to talk about," I asked him.

"Good food," he whispered.

"Good food?"

"Carrots and stuff," the boy said, looking away from me. "Bananas, peaches, apples," he added as though programmed.

"Do you like any of them?" I asked.

"No," he responded with the most emotion I had seen from him.

The child's food repertoire was quite extensive. He would eat cheeseburgers, pizza, spaghetti, hot dogs, ice cream, cake, milk, and soda pop. He used to eat chicken and broccoli—lots of the latter, his mother had indicated. Now, however, he would not eat any fruits or vegetables. If they were put on his plate, he would refuse to touch them. If his parents insisted, no matter how briefly, he would demonstrate his displeasure by screaming, thrashing, throwing the plate, and, occasionally, hitting his mother. I turned to the woman: "What do you want him to do?"

Without hesitating, "I want him to eat some fruit," she replied, then added, "not a lot, but some. I'm concerned about his health. Maybe I'm wrong, but his father's side of the family has a serious history of cardiac problems. I want my son to learn some good eating habits. Besides, the kids at school are making fun of him because he only brings peanut butter and jelly sandwiches. He won't ever bring an apple or banana to school."

I looked toward the boy. "Is that true?" He nodded. "Does it bother you that they are teasing you?" He nodded again. "If you ate fruit with your friends, they wouldn't bother you, is that right?"

"Yes," he said softly.

The problem was clearly one of compliance. The child was physically healthy. He was a bright, adorable, butch-haired blonde kid who was fine so long as he could eat what he wanted. Two years earlier, his noncompliance had centered around bedtime. He refused to go to bed when requested, and demanded that he be allowed to sleep with his mother and father. If his demands were not met, he would scream until his parents acquiesced. Present problems centered around following his mother's request. She shared, "Takes me 20-million times to ask him to do something. I start out soft, then I have to scream." She paused for a moment to place her hand on Corey's head. "He goes to bed fine now," she said.

"What did you and your husband do to change things?"

"We set up a routine, we were consistent, and we made sure he went to bed, screaming or not."

"How long did it take for your son to learn your expectations?" I asked.

"Only a few days," the woman replied.

I turned toward Corey, allowing the woman time for her private thoughts: "Tell me some of the things you like to do?" He named many activities, including swimming, bike riding, coloring, reading, TV, and playing with his friends. His reinforcers were varied and plentiful. I looked at his mother: "What do you suppose will happen if tonight, at dinner, you place on his plate a cheeseburger, some potato chips, and an inch-long, narrow strip of carrot? What will your son do?"

"He'll eat the cheeseburger first, then drink two glasses of milk if I let him, eat the chips, then get up and walk away from the table," she answered, smiling.

I faced the child: "Corey, what do you think you'll do with the food?" The child's voice was barely audible: "I'd eat the cheeseburger, drink some milk. . . . "

"Will you eat the potato chips?"

"Yes," he said.

"And the carrot?"

"Save it for another day," he replied with youthful wisdom. The child slumped into his mother's lap. Whimpering, he said to her, "I don't like to eat that stuff." She folded her arms around him; it appeared she was on the verge of crying.

"You don't have to do this, you know," I said to her. "At some point in the future, he'll eat fruits and vegetables. I assure you he's not the first child to grow up on cheeseburgers and peanut butter and jelly sandwiches. I do not think the problem is nutrition. I believe, clearly, the problem is one of compliance. I would suggest that you go home and talk with your husband about the importance of Corey following your requests. If you both agree that the time has come for your son to be more considerate of your wishes, the program will be a simple one. You will place a small piece of fruit, or carrot—your son's choice—on a plate. You will explain to him that he needs to eat what you have offered. You will discuss how important it is to help you by following your requests. You will then explain the contingencies: he will be able to go outside, play with his friends, watch TV, color, or whatever, as soon as the food is eaten."

She looked toward her son, then to me: "We have the same situation that we had with bedtime, don't we? Only the behavior has changed. My husband and I must make some decisions about his behavior, about his listening to us, about his willingness to cooperate. His eating isn't the problem?" she added more to herself. "I will call you later," she declared as she and her son walked from the office.

The call came an hour later. "We want to try your idea," the mother said to me. "Corey has chosen a piece of apple. He will stay in the house until he finishes it, is that correct?"

"Yes," I answered, then asked, "How big a piece of apple?"

"About the size of a dime," she indicated. I smiled.

The next call came after some 2 hours. I could hear the child screaming in the background. "Are all children this difficult?" the woman asked.

"Some, yes," I answered.

"He's screaming that he hates you and me and carrots and apples. It has started to rain and he is blaming me for that. I can't believe I am spending my day off listening to this child scream because I am asking him to eat one small bite of a peeled apple. But I'm half way there, I can sense it," she said with some confidence. "He's beginning to move closer to the apple."

"Stay with it," I urged. Twenty minutes later, the next phone call came. The child wanted to speak with me. For several minutes he complained about the apple's size, about how bad it would taste. He then asked me if he had to eat it. I urged him to finish the apple so he could play with his friends. I told him that his mom and dad believed it was very important for him to do as they wished; that he could help his mom and dad by eating that small piece of fruit.

One more call came—10 minutes after I had spoken with the boy. "He ate it!" Mother exclaimed. "He has the biggest smile on his face and he couldn't wait for me to call you and tell you that he had done it. He is very proud of himself. His crying stopped the moment he placed the apple in his mouth. He chewed it, swallowed it, then smiled from ear to ear. I think he feels that he really accomplished something important," she said with pride. "Tomorrow . . . a peach."

It was a start. It represented a family decision to work through a problem that had begun to cause difficulties for everyone, including the child. Come school time, the child would have an apple in his lunch box. That would make him feel better.

MARCIA

Notice which of the child's behaviors initially receives the most attention from her parents. Notice further the importance for remembering the power that cues have in setting the stage for behaviors, as well as the power that reinforcement contingencies have in influencing the occurrences of behavior. Lastly, observe the child's reaction when someone finally, firmly directs her behavior—in other words, tells her what not to do.

I was asked by the family's pediatrician to see the 20-month-old child after the youngster's mother began noticing an increase in gagging and vomiting that, upon examination, appeared to have no physiological base. I visited with the child and her parents during an evening meal at the family's home. The parents were requested to carry through with feeding their child as though I were not present.

The child sat comfortably in her high chair as Mother prepared her meal. My presence was barely noticed as she played quietly with toys that, I was told, always occupied a position beside the food on her tray. "We have the most problem with vegetables," Mother shared as she sat across from her daughter. "Fruits and meat are accepted without hesitation; but carrots, squash, and the like cause her to gag and sometimes vomit."

"You mean she gags and vomits when those foods are brought to her lips?" I clarified.

"Yes, almost always," the woman replied. "Often she will gag before they touch her tongue."

"But not with either the fruits or meats," I asked.

"Never," Mom answered as she looked toward her husband for verification.

"Never," Father echoed.

"Feed her the fruits and meats for a few moments," I requested. "I'd like to see her approach to the foods, her swallowing, and general reaction to being fed." As Mother had suggested, the child ate willingly when offered what she liked. Mom and Dad remained silent as the child swallowed. "Now the squash," I requested. The child's watchful eyes immediately saw what had been placed on the spoon. The filled spoon had yet to touch the child's lips when the gagging started. Mother retracted the spoon, waiting for the child to calm, then offered the spoon of squash once more. This time the child's gagging resulted in vomiting. The vomiting, in turn, was followed by crying. The child was immediately removed from the high chair and carried, while being consoled, into the kitchen, where she was cleaned. Mother than brought her back to the dinning room table, but rather than placing her daughter in the high chair, she held the child in her lap and finished feeding her the meats and fruits. When the jars were emptied, the child was lowered to the floor where her toys and books were located.

Mom turned to me. "Fruits and meats are fine. Anything else and she gets sick," the woman said.

I sat quietly for a few minutes, reviewing what I had seen. The child used the presence and absence of the meat, fruits, or vegetables to know whether to swallow or force a gag. While little commotion was paid to the child's desired eating, a great deal of attention was provided when the child vomited: she was removed from the chair, talked to soothingly, cleaned gently, rubbed around her forehead and cheeks, brought back to the table, placed on her mother's lap, provided with desired foods, and later allowed to play with her toys and games. She was also allowed to watch the squash as it vanished into the bottom of the kitchen sink. "I think it is necessary for you both to decide whether you want your daughter to show her displeasure with food choices by gagging and vomiting. Eating vegetables appears not to be the essential issue," I said to the parents. "Your daughter is not the only child who has developed food preferences and has figured out a way to let you know, rather clearly, the nature of those preferences. I would suggest that you discuss whether her choice of communication is acceptable to you. My guess is that if you withhold vegetables from her the vomiting and gagging will cease for the moment."

"But she might make herself vomit if she doesn't like a flavor of ice cream," Father said with some degree of sarcasm.

"Not totally out of the question," I responded.

"Are we doing something wrong?" Mother asked.

"Don't worry about that for the moment. I'll come back tomorrow night, and we'll develop a program," I said as I stood. "By the way, have you ever told Marcia not to gag or vomit?" I asked before walking out the front door.

The parents looked at one another. "I don't think so," Mom said as though such a possibility was hard to believe.

"The minute you see your daughter begin to gag, I want you to point your finger toward her and with a deep, sharp voice, say, 'No gag!'" I explained as I sat next to Mom and her daughter the following evening. "I also want you to immediately remove whatever toys are on the feeding tray. At the same time, let her know that you appreciate her more acceptable eating habits. Tell her how pleased you are when she swallows."

"We're giving her a lot of attention when she gags and vomits, aren't we?" Father asked as though he already knew the answer.

"Quite a bit, particularly in comparison to what happens when she doesn't gag. If, or when she vomits, tell her sharply that you are not pleased and continue feeding her as though nothing had happened."

"I shouldn't clean her?" Mom asked.

"Not right after it happens. Her vomiting starts a lengthy, somewhat complex chain of events that ultimately ends up allowing her to eat what she wants. Clean her after dinner is finished," I answered.

"Then I shouldn't hold her on my lap?"

"Preferably not during dinner; most assuredly not after vomiting."

"Then we have been doing things wrong," Mom reflected.

"Let's say you have been teaching your daughter that her vomiting will produce what she values. You will now teach her that her swallowing will produce that end. "

"So by cleaning her, soothing her, and bringing her to my lap after she's vomited, we've told her that vomiting is okay?"

"Perhaps not okay, but you told her what would happen when she vomited," I explained. "She doesn't get to be on your lap when she eats quietly, willingly. She has to vomit to get there," I suggested.

"I never thought about it that way," Mom replied.

"Few of us do," I answered supportively.

The child was given three spoonfuls of fruits before the squash was brought to her mouth. Predictably, she gagged when the vegetable reached her lips. Mother, unhesitatingly, placed the toys on the floor, moved toward her daughter and exclaimed, "We do not gag!" The child started, and tears came to her eyes. Mother winced, but took a deep breath and provided her daughter with a small spoonful of meat. "Thank you for swallowing," Mom said warmly as though the previous stern remark had never occurred. A small amount of squash was placed on the child's lips. Again the gag occurred. Again the firm admonition. Mother followed her remark with a second taste of squash then, almost simultaneously, a larger taste of fruit. The absence of gagging brought proclaimed appreciation from both Mom and Dad. The child smiled broadly; her tears disappeared as she basked in the clapping and verbal praise. There was no further gagging during the meal.

The following lunch session produced both a resurgence of gagging and one incident of vomiting. Mom repeated the "No gagging" demand and, as requested, removed the toys from the tray and continued feeding without cleaning the child. She treated the vomiting as though it had not happened. The child reacted with understandable surprise: a predictable routine had changed. A new one had begun, however: successful swallows, unaccompanied by gagging, vomiting, or complaints produced valued appreciation. The child often found herself sitting on her mother's lap after she had eaten her meals, which now consistently included a small amount of vegetables. The child's gagging and forced vomiting ceased by the end of the second week of intervention.

ROBERT

A brief, delightful case with a surprisingly common theme: a child dictating his choice of foods by declaring what he likes and doesn't like. Usually no big deal. In this instance, however, the child hadn't tried 99% of the foods he "didn't like." Accidentally, through his own words and his parents' literal interpretations of those words, the child's diet was limited and "boring." Notice the following familiar themes: neutrality and the "this first" contingency.

"He only eats plain yogurt, cheese and peanut butter crackers, and sliced apples," Mom explained over the phone. "Breakfast, lunch, and dinner," she added, clearly punctuating each word with a layer of personal frustration.

"How about fluids?" I asked.

"Milk and apple juice, as much as I will give him," she explained.

"Bring him to my university office, along with his favorites and some flavored yogurt, Pepperidge Farm (slightly salted) Goldfish, and some canned peaches or pears," I requested.

"What should I tell him when he asks where we're going with all that food he doesn't like?" Mom asked.

I couldn't tell whether she was serious or smiling. I smiled enough for both of us: "Tell him he's going to have a good time."

"He's not going to buy that," she stated with assurance.

The child was one of the most verbally precocious 4-year-old's I had ever met. If I hadn't known better, I would have thought I had gone to see him to learn about stellar bodies, dinosaurs, and (thankfully something I was familiar with) the Denver Broncos. When it came my turn to speak, I asked him what he had eaten for breakfast. "Apples, cheese and peanut butter crackers, and plain yogurt," he informed. When I asked him what he had for last night's dinner he stated, "Apples, cheese and peanut butter crackers, and plain yogurt." I didn't bother to ask him what he expected to have for lunch. "How about this?" I said, pointing to the blueberry-flavored yogurt.

"I don't like that," he responded stoically.

"This?" I asked, showing him the diced peaches.

"I don't like that either," he said equally impassively.

"Do you like this?" I asked showing him his plain yogurt.

"Yes, of course," he answered.

"This," I whispered, bringing a single Goldfish into plain view.

"I don't like that," he responded.

"Good," I answered as I placed it in my mouth. "Would you like your mom to stay in this room with us while you eat lunch?" He nodded.

I piled all the food onto the seat of a chair and brought it close to where the child was sitting. "What would you like first," I asked. He pointed to the apple. I cut a slice of apple into four parts and handed him one piece. "What next?" Cheese, peanut butter cracker. That was also divided into several pieces. He was given one. "Next?" He pointed to the plain yogurt. "You may have a taste of yogurt after you taste this," I said pointing to the flavored yogurt.

"I don't like that."

I turned to his mother: "Has he ever tried it?" I asked, in order to confirm what she had told me over the phone.

"No," she replied.

"What do you do when he says, 'I don't like that,'" I asked her.

"I say okay," she answered as though the response was obvious.

"Do you want him to try other foods?" I asked the woman loud enough so her son could hear.

"Of course," she responded.

I turned to Robert. "Would you like some plain yogurt?"

"Yes," he answered.

"You may have some after you have had a taste of this, this, or this," I said pointing to the Goldfish, the flavored yogurt, and the peaches, respectively.

"But I don't like them," he answered.

"Mom," I said, facing the woman, "would you leave us for a few moments. I'll come and get you in a second." The child watched nervously as his mother exited from the office. I quickly turned to the child. "Do you want your mom to be here?"

"Yes," he responded.

"Good, then take a little bite of one of these, then a taste of your yogurt, and I will get her."

"But I don't like them."

"You've never tasted them, Robert, so you don't even know what they taste like. Do you know what a scientist is?"

"Yes," he answered. "A scientist does experiments."

"Good," I responded. "Now, would you like me to feed you a small taste of this experiment or would you like to experiment yourself?" I asked firmly as I picked up a small plastic spoon. It was not an easy choice for the child. "Just a taste," I said as I touched the spoon's tip to the flavored yogurt. He took the spoon and placed the taste to his tongue. Immediately, he took a large spoonful of the plain yogurt. As promised, I brought his mother into the room. "What next?" I asked him.

"Cracker," he answered.

"Okay, you may have a bite of cracker after you try one of these," I reminded. He pointed to the flavored yogurt. I handed him the spoon. "It's good, yes?" I asked, after he swallowed half a spoonful.

He shrugged his shoulders in a "Yeah, it's okay, sorta."

Before he left the office, some 45 minutes after he and his mother had arrived, the flavored yogurt had become as valued as the other foods his mother had initially brought. As I walked with them to their car, I suggested to Mother that she not take everything her son said literally, at least not quite yet. "He may be saying a lot of things he's heard, but he's probably not understanding the importance of all the words. In the present context," I added, "he's limiting his own chances to taste lots of fun things." I indicated that the "I don't like that" verbal response may be okay after something has been tried, certainly not before.

Dinner that night was to include a few very small pieces of french toast, some flavored yogurt, and whatever else the child desired. Until his diet broadened a little, the child would have a choice of what to eat second. His mom would chose what he would eat first. His words of food preference would be given a little more credibility after he and his taste buds had dabbled in some small, gustatory experiments.

"S"

All things considered, the following represents the most difficult "behavioral" case I have been involved with (it is still in progress). The many problems will be evident. Notice the various components that were considered before the program was begun. Notice further the "data collection" factor that was incorporated to help determine whether any progress was being achieved. Such data collection com-

ponents are particularly essential any time an "unpleasant" factor is
incorporated within the employed treatment.

The child was brought to my attention through one of the hospital's social workers who had been trying to assist the young-ster's 25-year-old mother with the many problems she was facing. It had been discovered several months earlier that Mother suffered a regressive neuromuscular disorder that had begun to influence both her motoric and cognitive capabilities. Mother's trials in daily living were further complicated by the fact that her similarly aged husband was struggling with a personal history of alcohol abuse, which often left him incapacitated throughout the day: it was rare that he could help his wife care for their young daughter who, it happened, had her own burdens to bear. At 28 months of age, the child had just begun to exercise her budding ability to walk. She had yet to speak her first word. Two weeks after birth, the child was g-tubed due to poor sucking and appetite; the augmentative feeding regime had been maintained throughout the days ever since.

The medical team sat together to decide whether it was appropriate at the present time to intervene in behalf of the child and her family. The team realized that parental cooperation in the effort would be unlikely, perhaps despite both parents' felt desire to assist. Working with the child at her home, therefore, was not feasible: the parents would require constant supervision during each of the proposed five or six daily feeding sessions, and no services, private or otherwise, were available to afford such constant scrutiny. It was equally unlikely that the hospital's rehabilitation department would be able to free its therapists to supervise Mother and child, even if the youngster could be brought to the hospital for every meal for, what was projected to be, many weeks. Had the family's present living situation not been so serious, consideration would have been given to delaying, perhaps for a year or so, efforts to help the child overcome her eating difficulties. The social worker shared that in her judgment the present feeding problems were creating serious problems for both Mother and

child; that the required g-tube feedings, which Mother person-
alized as a sign of maternal failure, were placing severe stress on an
already faltering relationship between Mother and child. The social
worker urged that every effort be made to intervene now. Waiting,
she added, could be very detrimental to the entire family. The team
agreed. Two decisions were made immediately. First, the child
would be brought into the hospital as an inpatient to allow for
constant supervision of the feeding program and to allow for the
withholding of all g-tube feedings. She would be kept well hy-
drated but would not be fed augmentatively. Second, a successful
program would be achieved only when the child's eating had come
under the complete control of the environment's natural feedback
of pleasant taste and reduction of hunger. Given the problems at
home, artificial reinforcement systems would not likely prove lasting or effective. The child's physiological system would have to
become her strongest ally.

The child, however, had been g-tubed from near birth. She
had never experienced any consistent effort at "po" feeding; she
had never experienced any success with "po" feeding. Any hunger
the child experienced had been consistently and repeatedly re-
lieved through passive means: the child had taken no part in mol-
lifying any physical or emotional discomfort from hunger. Indeed,
there was a good chance the child had little knowledge of the
physical or emotional sensation of hunger. Not problematic was an
additional, highly complicating factor: while the child would swallow, although not consistently, her own saliva, she would not
swallow anything else. In fact, she had never swallowed any food
or liquid placed in her mouth. Her major avoidance response was a
soft, repetitive spitting: when food was placed on her tongue, she
would place the tip of her tongue into the soft tissue below her
lower lip, then she would blow air causing both her tongue and lip
to vibrate, creating a sound often joyous to a listening parent. In
"S's" case, there was little joy from the persistent activity; any food
or liquid placed on her tongue would be showered into the air.
Before any procedure could produce success, this avoidance response had to be worked through.

Exploration showed that the child was willing and capable of placing an empty spoon into her own mouth. Further, she was happy to feed anyone other than herself any substance that was placed on the spoon. While we wanted her to place a filled spoon into her own mouth and swallow what was provided, there was little reason to believe that she had any idea that this was a "normal" part of eating. For her, foods, spoons, swallows, and all other associative paraphernalia were intended for someone else. That belief system, of course, had to be altered. The child first had to know hunger. She then had to reduce that unpleasant sensation by her own actions. For both to happen, the child had to learn to swallow food and/or liquid.

She was taken to the hospital's toy "store" where she selected several items of interest. Once back in the room, she was placed in a high chair—the toys were placed on the tray. She sat comfortably in the chair and allowed an empty spoon to gently graze her cheeks and lips. The spoon, bare of contents, was not a problem. The spoon was dipped in applesauce, then banana pudding, then chocolate pudding, then strained plums, peaches, and pears. It mattered not: the spitting was constant and successful—nothing, not even the child's saliva, remotely approached the back of the child's mouth.

Despite the fact that the child had had virtually nothing to eat for some 60 hours, she would sit quietly in her high chair, play with her toys, and gently spit back any food touching her tongue.

It became apparent that any attempts at reinforcing some approximation to swallowing would not work—the avoidance response of spitting was too entrenched. Reluctantly, the decision was made to force a swallow. The child would earn brief time (15 seconds) with a valued object or activity once the swallow occurred. The procedure was as follows: the child would be held at a near 45-degree angle in a nurse's arms. A small quantity of baby food would be brought into the child's mouth. Care would be taken to "shake" the food from the spoon so that it would fall onto the back of the child's tongue. Every effort was made to avoid eliciting a gag. Occasionally, using a Brecht feeder, 1 or 2 cc's of liquid also would be placed near the back of the child's mouth, more near the cheek than tongue. Because of the forced component and the strong likelihood the child would find the approach uncomfortable, it was decided to keep track of the number of seconds that transpired between the time the food touched the tongue and the occurrence of the swallow. If the procedure was successful, the time period between the two events would decrease. The nurse holding the child would be in a perfect position to know exactly when the swallow occurred. As soon as it did occur, the child would be brought upright, provided with the toy of her choice, and the "swallow time" would be documented.

The child did not swallow the food fed to her. With remarkable skill, she pushed both food and liquid forward to the tip of her tongue. After a few seconds of spitting, her mouth was empty. The procedure required an additional component: the avoidance response of spitting would be prevented. Once the food was placed in the child's mouth, her lips would be held tightly closed by a nurse's or therapist's fingers. Any attempt at spitting would result in a forceful rebuke. Occasionally, using a Brecht feeder, liquid would be placed deep in the child's mouth to help elicit a swallow. Most often, the liquid would be added to the "solids" already in the mouth. Once the food was in the child's mouth, the individual holding the child's lips would quietly, rhythmically ask the child to swallow. The term "swallow" would be emphasized once the behavior occurred. If necessary, an additional person would try to soothe the child by softly rubbing the side of her cheek.

During the first trial with the lip-closure component, "S" held the food and liquid in her mouth, struggling to spit, for nearly 85 seconds before the first swallow occurred (likely her very first swallow of food in her entire life). Those in the private room erupted with excitement. The child was brought to an upright position. She appeared surprised by the clapping and verbal praise. The playing and "positive" feedback lasted some 15 seconds after which she was returned to the tilted position and food was placed in the back of her mouth. The process was repeated 11 additional times before the session ended. She was placed standing on the floor. We marveled at how quickly she walked from the room. The data showed that during the first set of 12 trials, the average time between food entering mouth and being swallowed was about 70 seconds. Anecdotal notes indicated that the child's struggling had gradually increased with each trial. By the end of the session, she was flushed and perspiring. It had been a difficult session for everyone.

By the end of the second full day of trials (six sessions of roughly 12 to 15 trials each were held throughout the day), the child's protesting surprisingly decreased to near nothing. She would whimper slightly upon seeing the spoon, but she would allow it to enter her mouth. Average time of swallowing had been reduced to near 45 seconds. During the first session on the third day, the occupational therapist who participated in the feeding session reported that the first seven swallows each occurred within an average of 15 seconds. The quick progress was short-lived: by the afternoon of that day, the child's struggling intensified to a level far surpassing that of the first day. Average swallow time was well over a minute. The procedure was quickly evaluated, but only the "reinforcement" component was changed. The child was now seated in a wheelchair. She enjoyed being taken for rides around the floor. The new reinforcement contingency: swallow and take a ride. No other changes were made after looking closely at the data. Progress was occurring. The child, after all, was working through a process that she had been used to for nearly her entire life. It was important to be patient and continue in a consistent fashion. The goal was to teach the child the new process: nice things happen when you swallow. Such a lesson, we realized, would take time.

The evening trials were much more successful: less struggling; swallowing occurring after some 20 to 30 seconds. (The child's overall body weight had dropped about 4%. The physician decided to augmentatively feed the child during the evening. She was given roughly 40% of her normal daily caloric intake; the belief was that this additional intake would not disturb the procedure.) By the fourth day of treatment, the struggling had nearly ceased. More critically, there were times when the child no longer required anyone to hold her lips closed. On those occasions, the feeder could gently remove his or her fingers from the child's lips and quietly remind the youngster not to spit while gently rubbing her cheeks and forehead. The child would sit still, often holding her head at an upward angle. During about a third of those trials she would make a semi-swallow: any food toward the back of the mouth would be swallowed; food still at the front of the mouth would not be swallowed—the child would allow it to drool from her mouth. The semi-swallows were seen as big successes. The child was experiencing the feeling from swallowing something substantive. It was a strong beginning.

The procedure continues. It has been in operation for only 1 week—a relatively short time compared to the number of weeks the child learned not to eat by mouth. All expectations are that the child will continue showing progress. The "half" swallows are the keys to showing the child that she can influence her own hunger. That cognitive realization will not occur tomorrow. It will, however, happen.

(*Progress note:* On the first day of the second week of treatment, "S" consumed 2-1/2 ounces of banana pudding. She took 18 swallows. There was no spitting. According to the occupational therapist who fed the child, "'S' opened her mouth when the spoon approached her lips. The child was relaxed throughout the 30-minute session. She was required to take three swallows of food before receiving any reinforcement. The beginning of self-feeding was initiated. I held the child's dominant hand in mine. Together we scooped some pudding and brought it into her mouth. She did not fight me at all." The therapist, with his typical manner of understatement suggested, "With luck she'll like feeding herself." He concluded, "Excellent session.")

DAVID

A good example showing that poor feeding, again, is often related to other behaviors. Notice the use of various "management" techniques to help a child not only give up a plastic nipple, but also to become a little more considerate of his parents' wishes.

This child ate just fine so long as his food was provided through a bottle. At 24 months of age, he had never willingly accepted any food substances from a cup, spoon, or any similar utensil. Mom and Dad had been unknowingly taught to puree any number of tasty dishes and to squeeze them into a bottle. They had also been taught to allow their son to stay up later in the evening than either wished; taught how to retract a request that their son chose not to comply with; taught any number of other "small" issues that seemed to work in the son's favor. Who was the teacher? David. What were his teaching tools? Tantrums. His future looked bright. His present was somewhat more suspect.

The initial call came from the child's maternal grandmother. She and her daughter had read somewhere that a child who refuses to give up a bottle before the age of 3 is likely emotionally insecure, immature, and perhaps disturbed. "Comfortable and quite satisfied with the bottle would be a more accurate characterization," I suggested to the woman. "While Mom and Grandma might be a little disturbed, child is likely doing fine." The woman and I spoke for several minutes, during which it became apparent that the youngster had discovered that whenever any effort was made to have him put away the bottle in favor of a spoon, his highly vocal tantrums would always result in the effort's rapid termination. It was further evident that Mom and Dad had failed to reach a consensus as to whether the bottle should or should not be retired. I suggested that the family bring the child to the hospital, where I could try some things with him while the adults viewed from behind a one-way mirror. It turned out I didn't get a chance to do anything but listen briefly to the youngster scream. I had no more sat him in a high chair and brought a bowl of pudding beside his bottle then he began to scream clamorously. Removing the pudding from the tray failed to dampen his protesting. I could not redirect him or calm him with my voice or what toys I had brought into the room. He was "on," and I held to the notion that he would only be satisfied (and quieted down) if he saw me flush the pudding down a porcelain facility. I stood up from my chair and walked behind the one-way mirror, requesting that his mother join us in the examination room. The child quieted and reached his arms out as soon as he saw his mother. "Is this typical of him?" I asked the woman as she held her child.

She shared that he screamed whenever she tried to feed him with a spoon. Then she added, "He also screams when it is time for bed, time to bathe, or time to do most anything he doesn't want."

I sat with the family for a few moments talking mainly about what expectations they had for their son. It was apparent that Mom and Dad had never had a serious discussion about each other's values and preferences regarding David's behavior. I requested that they do some "homework" for me and that when it was completed to call me. I further suggested that at the moment they not concern themselves with how David eats. "Give him the bottle," I said.

The homework involved three major components. The first item dealt with their son's behaviors. They were asked to consider what each wanted David to do and not to do around bedtime, bathtime, and while eating. The parents were urged to privately decide what each considered to be desired and undesired behaviors. (The determined behaviors were called "behavior pairs.") I explained to the parents that for David to understand their expectations, the expectations had first to be determined then communicated clearly and consistently. The second item was a request to have the parents run a daily log of their reactions to David whenever he manifested either a determined desired or undesired behavior. In other words, they were to write down what they did whenever David behaved desirably or otherwise. I explained that their son's behavior was greatly impacted by the reactions it received; that if David discovered that his tantrums brought him something he valued, then the tantrums would be repeated in the future. The third item requested that they note how David responded to their reactions. The parents were to determine what effects, if any, their feedback was having on their son's behaviors. Did he seem to like or dislike what they did? The next time I saw them, the parents handed me a five-page report indicating what had happened over the past 4 days. It was readily apparent that son David was running the house. It was equally obvious that neither parent was pleased with their present circumstances. The decision was made and agreed upon to put aside the feeding issue for a short while. The first order of business was to show David that his tantrums would no longer enable him to avoid the tasks his parents believed were necessary. Secondly, it was necessary to show the youngster how some alternative behaviors on his part could bring him much of what he valued.

After looking at the diary's entries together, the parents realized that David's tantrums were producing effects he desired: the tantrums helped him delay bedtime, avoid taking a bath, and control other activities that included eating only from a bottle. By giving in to the tantrums, the parents were unwittingly teaching David to have tantrums more frequently and under more varied conditions. The data regarding bedtime were particularly illuminating. The child had tantrums each evening when first put to bed. The parents had allowed David to scream for varying amounts of time (ranging from 20 to 30 minutes) before removing him from his bedroom and allowing him to stay with them until he fell asleep in their arms. Rather than learning to go to bed as requested, David was learning to cry more intensely in order to be with his parents. Because both parents were particularly upset with their son's evening behavior, I suggested that they target their efforts on bedtime. The process was not too complicated. They first had to mutually agree upon what time the child would be placed in bed. Next, they were asked to develop a predictable routine so David could determine that bedtime was near—that there would be time for relaxation, stories, games, and the like, but that when the appointed hour arrived, bedtime meant bedtime. David would be allowed to tantrum for as long as he chose. David cried nearly 65 minutes the first evening. The crying was slightly longer the second night. He cried for 5 minutes the third night and did not whimper the fourth night. The following morning, the child was told how pleased his parents were that he went to bed so nicely. He was given a special treat at breakfast, and after being told once more how pleased his parents were that he went to bed "nicely," he was read an extra story that evening. When he went to bed without fussing after the extra story, Mom commented, "Bribery sure works." I spent several minutes explaining that what they were doing had nothing in common with bribery. The parents didn't seem to be concerned about the semantic issues. They were pleased with the results.

Cooperative bathing, diaper changing, and complying with type-one requests produced equally positive feedback. David was beginning to understand that his desired behaviors would result in his parents' warm attention and recognition. He was also learning that his tantrums were no longer as effective as they once had been. That lesson was essential, for he was soon to be asked to eat food with a spoon.

His tantrum began the moment he noticed the bowl of pudding that rested beside his bottle. Without words, Mother removed him from the high chair and placed him in his bed. David remained there until he was quiet for 30 seconds. (His loud tantrum, that grew suddenly milder once in his room, lasted less than 4 minutes.) He was returned to his high chair. He was given a small taste of food from his bottle. It was important for him to know that the bottle was not going to be removed. Mother placed an empty spoon in his mouth then followed its retraction with the bottle. The bottle was removed and placed alongside the bowl of pudding. "Taste this," Mother said, showing David the chocolate pudding, "then you can have your bottle. If you cry, you will go to your room." David did cry and was once again removed to his room. He stopped crying the moment Mother left him alone. After 30 seconds, she returned him to the high chair. David chose not to drink anything from the bottle. He was removed from the high chair. Mother stayed somewhat distant from him for the next hour. He was then returned to the high chair, the bottle, and the chocolate pudding. It would not be until nearly 4 hours later that the child would take the small amount of pudding from the spoon. Immediately, he was given the bottle. Before the day had ended, David had eaten over a dozen spoonfuls of pudding, each of which were followed by a drink from his bottle. His eating from a spoon soon included such delights as mashed potatoes, small pasta noodles, and much of what had been provided through the bottle. (The bottle, of course, was still available. It had, however, lost some of its popularity.) A week after the first bedtime bout, David ate his first raisin. A milestone of sorts.

BERTA

A good review of alternative feeding methods available for an infant who appears ambivalent about drinking from a bottle. Notice how the "experiment" with the pacifier helped to determine whether the child was experiencing physical distress from eating. Please note: this case was carefully supervised by a pediatrician. The techniques should not be replicated without approval from a child's attending physician.

The premature baby's corrected age was nearly 4 months when I saw her. I sat on the floor with the child, her mother, and speech and physical therapists. Although the family's pediatrician was not at hand, she was well aware of the procedures I would use to assist the youngster and her parents. The chief concern centered around the child's typical unwillingness to consume much more than an ounce of formula at any given meal. I was also informed that once the child stopped drinking, she would often become quite "angry" (she would scream and arch her back—signs that I had come to associate with possible physical discomfort). When I asked if the child had been thoroughly examined for possible contraindications to "po" feeding, the therapist said the child hadn't. The therapist indicated that the pediatrician felt the child was not experiencing any particular distress from eating. (The child's lungs were clear, and there had been no history of choking, gagging, or turning blue during feeds.) However, the physician wanted to know whether I sensed that additional examinations were warranted.

The professionals and I watched the child carefully as Mother fed her formula from a bottle. The child stopped her sucking after consuming about 20 ccs (less than an ounce) of food. Immediately, the child began screaming and arching her back. "What do you usually do when this begins to happen?" I asked Mother.

"I give her the pacifier," Mom answered. "It's the only way I can calm her down."

"Try the bottle once more," I asked. The therapists and I watched the child's small tongue work hard to push the nipple from her mouth. Mom picked up on the child's effort and removed the bottle. The screaming and arching began in earnest. "How long has she been doing this?" I inquired.

"Nearly a month," Mom replied.

"And if you give her the pacifier, she will stop?" Mother smiled, nodded, and placed the pacifier into the child's mouth. The screaming and arching ceased immediately. "Try the bottle once more," I asked. The child swallowed a few drops more, then pushed the nipple away. Again the screaming returned. The pacifier was returned to the child.

"Weird?" the young mother asked.

"She's telling us something," I said touching the child's cheek, "I'm just not sure of her message. We'll try a few things."

One of the therapists returned with a small jar of sweet potatoes and a makeshift Brecht feeder. Despite the fact that the child quieted when provided the pacifier, I was still concerned that perhaps she was hurting somewhat from swallowing the food. She hadn't eaten in several hours, yet after consuming only a few ccs of food she seemed quite content to simply suck on her pacifier. My intention was to feed her more and observe whether she would cry and arch her back. If she remained calm during and after feeding, then the screaming and arching might be behavioral rather than organic. The opposite could also be possible. As a side issue, I wanted to see if she would eat by some means other than the nippled bottle. Maybe the message behind her behaviors was, "Hey, I'm still hungry."

A small spoonful of sweet potatoes was placed in the child's mouth. Her small tongue worked the food back until it was comfortably swallowed. She was given a few ccs of formula and that too was swallowed without incident. Mother was asked to give the child her pacifier even though the youngster was quiet. I explained that since it was essential to determine whether the child's screaming was reflective of physical pain or the desire for the pacifier, it was important to provide the pacifier at times other than when the child was screaming. In that way, the screaming might reduce itself sufficiently to give all of us a better picture of the purpose behind the screaming.

The pacifier was removed and another spoonful of sweet potatoes was provided. More formula was also provided through the Brecht feeder. The child swallowed and remained quiet. The pacifier was returned to the child. "Let's see what happens with the bottle," I said to Mother. "When you remove the pacifier, give the child her bottle. If she screams, do not give her the pacifier. Instead, give her a little sweet potato and formula through the syringe. If she quiets, we're in 'fat city.'" Mother looked toward me. "I mean we'll have a good handle on what is going on," I explained apologetically.

The child sucked for a short while, then she began screaming after pushing the bottle's nipple from her mouth. She immediately quieted when given a spoonful of sweet potatoes, followed by a few ccs of syringed formula, followed by her pacifier. As her pediatrician had predicted, the child's screaming appeared unrelated to any physical discomfort from eating. For reasons known only to the youngster, she simply wasn't fond of the nippled bottle. She was, however, quite fond of food. Before the session ended, she consumed roughly 60 ccs of food and liquid. She consumed some 70 ccs the following meal. She remained pleasantly comfortable and quiet throughout the latter feeding. Mother was asked to consult both her pediatrician and a dietitian to learn which foods would be best for the small infant.

LAURA

Notice the new term—"baseline." When using artificial reinforcement to develop, increase, or maintain "po" feeds, a baseline measure is an essential addition. Notice also how the child's values and

> *interests were incorporated in the reinforcement program. This example will provide a simple way of charting progress. Often the charting will prove very reinforcing to the child.*

I met the delightful 7-year-old and her parents in my office. Mother had called earlier indicating a perpetual problem with her daughter's eating habits. The bubbly, affectionate youngster had experienced a series of gastrointestinal difficulties from birth, along with other physical setbacks that had produced the near total loss of vision in one eye and a persistent problem with fine-motor tasks. Nothing that she had endured, however, had dampened either her spirit, intelligence, or determination to get as much joy out of life as possible. The present problem clearly indicated that eating food was not an activity that contained such pleasure. "I eat," she said expressively with a huge smile and a high-pitched tone, when I asked her about her eating habits.

"Not much," her father said lightly.

"Oh, Dad," the youngster exclaimed as she smacked his shoulder affectionately, "I eat."

She was as skinny as a proverbial rail, but healthy. She couldn't have weighed more than 30 pounds soaking wet and carrying two bags of sand. (I later called the child's gastroenterologist, who suggested that a few extra pounds wouldn't hurt the child and would no doubt help the concerned parents.)

We spent the remainder of our time together developing a procedure to help the child eat just a little more. I sensed that whatever methods I suggested would be effective because the child seemed quite taken by me and appeared more than willing to follow my requests. (I knew I was liked because I too was the recipient of two affectionate smacks to the shoulder.)

The family and I first developed a "reinforcement menu" that reflected the child's important interests and values. Laura shared that she liked TV, going outside to be with friends, playing games with Dad, helping Mom clean the house, and bowling. I explained that I wanted the child to have both immediate, positive feedback for eating, as well as a few moderately long-range, equally positive goals to shoot towards. The child's reinforcement menu provided options for both.

The parents were requested to keep track of the number of swallows of solid food the child would consume during each meal for the next 3 days. The total number of swallows would be added and averaged for each of the days. (The lunch meal's tabulations were taken by the child's teacher, who was more than willing to offer his assistance.) The calculated average number of swallows would serve as a baseline upon which future reinforcement, chosen from the menu, would be determined. (Without knowing the baseline of swallows, we might have asked the child to eat too much or too little. We wanted her to succeed, but we also wanted her to gain a couple of pounds.) The parents called a week after our initial meeting. We met in my office to review the baseline data and to set up the reinforcement component of the procedure. The swallowing data were quite consistent: the child averaged roughly 20 swallows of food per meal. We decided to plot the "per meal swallows" on a chart so the child could see how well she was doing. She would be given the opportunity to fill in the chart. A line graph was drawn depicting the days of the week on the bottom (horizontal) line and the numbers 0 through 50 (representing possible swallows) on the vertical line. It looked something like this:

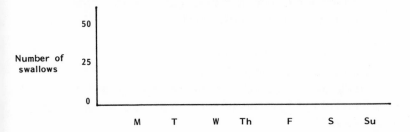

We then plotted the number of swallows Laura averaged per meal: Monday (the first day the baseline data were recorded) she had 18 swallows for breakfast, 21 for lunch, and 23 for dinner. The three meals averaged 20.6 swallows. (We dropped the .6.) A blue star was drawn above the "M" (for Monday) approximately across from where the number "20" would be written. Tuesday, Laura again averaged 20 swallows per meal. Again, a blue star was drawn above the "T" (for Tuesday), roughly where the number "20" would be located on the horizontal line. This process continued for the third day the baseline data were taken.

With the data and chart in hand, I met with the child to explain how the procedure would work. The astute youngster nearly beat me to the punch. "I have to eat that many bites every meal before I can watch TV, go outside, or go bowling, right?"

"Almost," I answered. "For you to go outside, watch TV, help Mom around the house, you must eat that many bites. But if you want to go bowling or see a movie . . . "

"Or rent a movie?" she asked.

" . . . Or rent a movie, you must eat at least one extra bite per meal. "

"A big bite?" she inquired hesitantly.

"No, just an extra bite," I assured her, which produced an exaggerated sigh of relief. "Each extra bite will provide you with a bonus star. You and your parents will decide how many bonus stars you will need to go bowling or see a movie."

"And if I don't take any extra bites?"

"That's okay, it's your choice."

"And if I don't eat at least the same amount as I did before?"

"Bad news," I answered quickly, smiling. "Can't watch TV. . . . "

"Or go outside," she added.

"Or lots of other things," I said.

"So I'll eat the same amount, maybe a little more." She paused for a moment. "If I get lots of bonus stars, can we all go out for Dairy Queen?"

"You want me to go with you?" I asked.

"Yes," she replied excitedly.

"You bet," I stated.

Dairy Queen was added to the menu. Two weeks later, the child, her three cousins and I went for Dairy Queen. She had gained only 6 ounces in those 2 weeks. At least she hadn't lost any weight, and that was seen as a good start. It would require almost 12 months before she had put on the desired 2 pounds. Perhaps not an overly impressive amount of gain by some standards, but in this child's case, the child's parents were thrilled.

"JP"

A good case to end on. Mom forgot that kids are different. She expected her son's eating behavior to be similar to that of her daughter's. I doubt it works that way too often.

The gutsy little 6-month-old boy, born 6 weeks prematurely, with a whole lot of physical problems, greeted me with a delightful smile when our eyes first fell upon one another. The major problem: after initially gaining nearly an ounce a day, inexplicably no weight gain had occurred for several months. The family's pediatrician could find no physiological explanation for the change. Conversation with Mom and Dad revealed that the breast-feeding child would appear satisfied after drinking only a few ounces from Mom. She felt he might be losing interest in breast feeding. Dad indicated that he had had some success with spoon feeding small amounts of cereals to the child during the late evening hours. All in all, it appeared as though the child was eating less than previously, which may have accounted for the absence of weight gain. Although the child had been fed somewhat earlier, I suggested that Dad try feeding the child solids. Typical of an exploration session, I wanted to watch whatever problems the child would experience eating from a spoon.

Happily, there were no problems. The child consumed very willingly roughly 4 ounces of cereal and bananas for his main meal, 1 to 2 ounces of banana pudding for dessert, and a few drops of Mom's milk that were given via a spoon. The family and I went into their living room. Mother and Dad, as you might expect, were elated over their child's eating. I referred them to a dietitian to gain information about caloric intake, but beyond that there was little I had done or little that needed doing. Almost apologetically, Mom explained, "I never thought he was hungry. He never tells me he's hungry. I expect a cry or something as a sign that it's time to eat. My daughter," she continued, "would howl the moment she would awaken. If food wasn't forthcoming immediately, she'd let me know. I guess I expected 'JP' to be like her. Same Mother and Father. Same house. But he's not like his sister. She used to scream. He sits and quietly waits," she chuckled, as she hugged her child warmly.

CHAPTER ELEVEN

Influencing a Child's Behavior

Certainly much of the material found here came from research findings and theoretical tenets of others who often spoke of children's behavior in general. Yet an equal amount, indeed more of the critical material, came from the kids who sat across from me and unabashedly shared their private and public "person." It was from these kids that the tenets and findings were reviewed and sometimes verified; from them that modifications in procedural thoughts and actions were attempted, remodified and replicated. I'd like now to touch upon a few findings and views that will offer you a notion of the foundation upon which the book's material was built, as well as provide additional thoughts for you to consider, specifically about your child's eating and generally about your child's behavior.

To Be Born Strong Willed

"She's so stubborn, so strong willed," Berta's mother said to me as her child arched her back and turned red with emotion. "This child was born with a temper hot enough to curdle milk. Is she ever going to change?" the woman asked as she placed the pacifier into the youngster's mouth. "Am I always going to need one of these," she mused, pointing to the weathered prosthesis.

More than a few of us would love to know if little Berta was indeed born with a temper hot enough to curdle milk or, for that matter, a disposition sweet enough to soothe the most stressed parent. Truth is, we aren't certain what personality or temperament trait any child is born with. Quickly, that's not because they aren't born with any emotional predispositions; it's because we aren't too good at figuring out their emotional expressions, and they aren't too good at expressing whichever emotions they may feel at the moment. Predictably, there's much we don't know about what infants have been given at the moment of conception and that which they have acquired by means of time's hands. Still, there are things we know (or think we know) about the "personality" traits infants bring with them as they enter our world.

1. No two children are ever exactly alike. Two children from the same family, living under the same roof, eating the same food and wearing the same clothes can be as different as the seasons of the year. What each possesses, what each will be, how each will act, can never be known by watching one and predicting to the other.

2. The infant is likely born with the ability to feel any number of different emotions. The infant may be predisposed to be aggressive or passive, hyper or hypo. The infant may be preset toward lover, lawyer, or laureate. Unfortunately, he can't tell us. For the time being, we can only speculate.

3. We know that little kids differ behaviorally and emotionally from birth. Enough differences have been observed among neonates to enable them to be graded as "easy" and "anything but easy." Of course, the grading process is a little suspect. Ultimately, parents must determine what constitutes each "characterization"; that judgment is likely to be made on the basis of how the parent feels when waking up in the morning.

4. We know that neonates come into the world with certain innate strengths—they have reflexes that appear designed to help them survive: touch an infant's cheek, and he will

turn toward the stimulus, take it into his mouth, and begin to suck. He'll try to walk even though he can't support himself, and he will try to swing his arms out then bring them together if he senses he's falling or losing support. Understatedly, all valuable, innate gifts.

5. We know that newborns can detect the difference between two notes only a step apart on a musical scale; know that they are capable of sensing and differentiating the tastes sweet and salty; know they will show specific sucking patterns when different substances are placed on their tongues—that when a sweet fluid is given every time the infant sucks, the baby will increase the sucking rate and take shorter rest periods than when no sweet substance is delivered; we know that even during the early days of life, newborns are sensitive to various smells and quickly learn to discriminate between the odor of their mother's breast pad and that belonging to another woman. And more. They can react to stimuli such as gentle touch and, only 2 hours old, they will follow a moving light with their eyes if the speed of the light is not too fast. They can flex and extend their arms and legs, smack their lips, and chew their fingers.[1]

6. We know infants are not blank pages, that their gestational life can dramatically influence their postnatal life.

7. We know that the neonate is an adaptive individual with the ability to learn from perhaps "breath one."

Learning and Self-Directed Behavior

Ironically, it is the infant's ability to learn at the earliest of ages (literally within hours of birth, if not before) that makes Berta's mom's assertion that her daughter was born angry so much more difficult to determine. By all observations, Berta appeared quite ticked when arching her back, screaming, and turning a light shade of red. But was the child born with the capacity to feel anger? Was her ability to express her emotions innate or learned? These are tough questions that have intrigued researchers, poets, and parents for eons.

> The exact time when emotions first appeared in human beings has long been a controversial topic. In 1919 John B. Watson, the behaviorist, claimed that infants are born with three major emotions—love, rage and fear. . . . But investigators who tried to confirm these theories had trouble identifying babies' emotional states. [Some researchers] concluded that emotional states are generalized in infants and not nearly so specific as [researchers] had believed. K. M. B. Bridges, writing in the Journal of Child Development over a half century ago, noted the difficulty in determining innate emotional states and concluded that newborns show only one emotion, an undifferentiated excitement (later termed "distress"), and that babies' emotions differentiate as they grow older, proceeding from the general to the specific. In short, babies may, from an early age, have a wide range of emotions that they cannot express specifically or that we cannot identify with certainty.[2]

Our interest in an infant's genetic predispositions toward certain emotions, traits, temperaments, and the like is certain not to wane. Perhaps one day, the little ones will get better at expressing what's going on inside their small bodies and/or we'll get better at identifying what they are "saying" and feeling during the hours immediately after birth. For the time being, Berta's asserted innate state of the specific emotion labeled "anger" is still problematic.

What is not problematic, however, is Berta's innate ability to learn. Clear evidence tells us that Berta's behavior is capable of being influenced by her internal (bodily) and external (surrounding) environments from the very moment she exits from the womb. Psychologist Dr. Fitzhugh Dodson has stated rather pointedly that a baby begins to learn from the moment she is born.[3] Researchers Lewis Lipsitt, Herbert Kaye, and Joseph Bosack have demonstrated infants' ability to learn at ages varying from 2 to 4 days.[4] Researchers Anthony DeCasper and William Fifer also showed the learning ability of 3-day-old infants.[5] For our purposes, what these and other studies suggest is that very young infants possess the ability to learn to do things, to behave in specific ways that bring them what they value. Said slightly differently, the infant has the ability to adapt to her environment and to learn from her environment. The noted developmental psychologist Jean Piaget believed strongly that infants possess the ability to adapt and, further, that they could continually modify their own behavior on the basis of their earliest experiences. They could, according to Piaget, learn to respond differently to different situations.[6] Perhaps in a most rudimentary sense, the infant's ability to adapt, to self-modify behavior, to learn to behave differently depending upon the conditions present, tells us that the infant has the ability, at a very early age, to begin becoming "self-directed"— that the infant, from the start, can begin to process experiential information; he can begin to learn and privately say, "When I do A, B happens; when I do C, D happens." So long as I'm taking the license to push things beyond what we know, perhaps the infant has the ability to begin making choices, that, again from the start, the infant's behavior can be seen as having purpose—"By damn," the little one says to himself at the ripe age of 72 hours, "when I do A (sleep), B happens (everyone leaves the room); when I do C (make some noise then suck), D happens (I get held and Mom allows me to feed—wow!). Frankly, my dear," the precocious one continues, "I much prefer the outcome of D. It is so stimulating. B stands for boooooring. Therefore, 'till something better comes along, I will continue doing C instead of A. Hey, Mom, I'm doing C," the little one quietly shouts, "bring on D."

Behavior Is Affected by the Feedback It Receives

While the above neonatal monologue is little more than enjoyable speculation, my experiences with many of the children seen and spoken of through this book suggest that their ability to learn, to make choices, to act purposively in order to gain access to what is valued does not require too many ticks of the maturational clock to come into existence. Jesse was only slightly older than 365 days when he began to experience pain when eating. It required only two handfuls of days beyond that for him to stop eating. His behavior was adaptive; it was purposive; it was intended to bring him what he valued: an absence of pain that occurred when he swallowed and digested his food. Neither his parents nor physicians were pleased with his choice of adaptation, but Jesse clearly did what he had to to take care of himself. Carly was half Jesse's age when she acquired her steadfast preference for her nanny's feeding approach over that of her parents. Her screaming, head turning, and thrashing were adaptive and purposive: she wanted nanny seated across from her, and she learned how to accomplish that end. Young Berta, despite being less than 4 months of age, knew how to communicate her disapproval of the bottled nipple. Her arching and screaming, too, were adaptive. She may have been angry; her anger may have been predisposed or learned, innate or acquired. Either way, her behavior had meaning and purpose, and it acquired such properties long before the child spoke her first word or attempted her first step.

Berta's ability to learn, to be influenced by her environment at the youngest of ages, should provide us with reasons for both excitement and trepidation. That the infant can be influenced tells us that we will begin to influence what she does, how she feels about what she does, how she feels about herself and feels about others, perhaps from the first time we hold her in our arms. That likelihood is cause for excitement and slight apprehension, for it reminds us that to best help the child and ourselves, it would be wise to have a sense of what we are doing when approaching the child. This latter point is especially true if Berta is a food refuser or manifests behavior problems that interfere with eating.

The logical question that flows from the above is, "How does Berta learn her unique, adaptive, purposive behaviors?" While several variables influence the child's cognitive systems, one appears especially critical for the child who has an eating difficulty, namely the type of feedback the child receives from her immediate environment. Let's do a quick review of some essential issues pertaining to feedback.

Internal and External Feedback

Feedback can be thought of as emanating from two sources: inside and outside our bodies. Both kinds of feedback are very familiar to you; both can dramatically influence what we (or our children) do. Let's try a couple of examples for both types.

A. You are a little careless when opening a letter. Your finger slips across the edge of the paper. You bleed. You hurt.
B. You spend hours working on a paper. When finished, you feel a great sense of joy and accomplishment for both your effort and the product.
C. On the way home from the concert you run a stop sign. You receive a $35.00 ticket, four penalty points, and a tongue lashing.
D. When you arrive home your child runs to you with an enormous hug.

A and B—inside (internal) feedback. C and D—outside (external) feedback. The feedback from the first two come from within your body—pain and joy. The feedback from the last two are, in a sense, given to you by someone else—the policeman, your child. Both types are important. *Point to remember: our own bodies can give us feedback; anyone (or any thing) we come in contact with can do the same.*

Positive and Negative Feedback

All of us will work hard to obtain positive feedback; all of us will work hard to avoid negative, or aversive, feedback. Let me say the last part in a slightly different way. If something we do produces positive feedback, we'll do again (in the near or distant future) what produced the positive feedback. Conversely, if something we do produces aversive, or negative, feedback, we won't repeat our actions, if such is possible. Let's quickly put these issues of internal/external and positive/negative feedback together.

Case A: Jack's esophagus and stomach hurt when he eats. He stops eating.

Feedback:

Internal. The felt pain is emanating from Jack's stomach and esophagus.
Negative. Jack does not like to hurt. The feedback (from his perspective) is negative.
Adaptive behavior. Jack will learn how to avoid the negative feedback. He will stop eating.

Case B: Pam has recently begun eating from a spoon. When she swallows, her mom smiles and tells her that she is very proud of her daughter's efforts.

Feedback:

External. The feedback is being provided by Mom, a source "outside" Pam.
Positive. Pam enjoys her mother's feedback. It is very positive.
Adaptive behavior. Pam will continue to swallow from a spoon. She enjoys pleasing her mother.

No Universal Definitions

What is viewed as positive feedback by one child may be viewed negatively by another. While nearly all infants and children will work hard to avoid feedback they perceive as pain, not all will respond in a similar manner to words intended to convey thanks; touches to the skin intended to show affection: gold, blue, or red stars intended to show appreciation; being sent to a room to "think" about transgressions; losing access to TV; or having the opportunity for earning an ice-cream cone. What is positive or negative is defined by, decided by, the individual who is receiving the feedback.

Quick Summary

Hence, behavior is affected by its consequences; it is affected by the feedback it receives. Also, a child will be more likely to repeat a behavior if that action produces feedback she perceives as positive. (Berta will willingly and continually swallow sweet potatoes if she likes the taste of sweet potatoes.) On the other hand, a child will be less likely to repeat a behavior if that action produces feedback she perceives as negative or aversive. (Berta will not continue to suck from a nippled bottle if her sucking is uncomfortable, unpleasant, or aversive.) Moreover, it is the child who determines the value of the environment's feedback; the child decides the value of sweet potatoes. Furthermore, since we provide some of the environmental feedback the child receives, it is understatedly wise to know what type of feedback we are providing, what behavior we are influencing, and what behavioral outcome our feedback is producing. Said slightly differently, we need to know what we are teaching our child to do. By sheer accident, purely unintentionally, we may be teaching the child to do the exact opposite of what we intend. Such actions may begin to impact the child's eating, as well as other essential behaviors. Notice the following examples demonstrating how the environment can inadvertently influence behavior.

Behavior Pairs

KAYLA

Note three issues: (1) the child's behavior, (2) the environment's reaction to the behavior, and (3) the probable results of the interaction.

Kayla is playing with her younger brother. She wants the toy he has in his hand. She whines and says, "Give me the toy." Her brother turns and hides the toy. Kayla whines louder. Mom becomes upset with all the noise. She walks to its source. She tells her son to give Kayla the toy.

Analysis: Kayla receives what she wants after she whines . . . and whines louder. Good chance the next time she doesn't get what she wants, she'll try whining . . . loudly.

Behavior	Environment's reaction	Results
Whining	Receives toy	Increase in whining when failing to get what she wants

---

KYLE

Again notice the same three components. In this example, there is an additional variable that warrants our attention. The variable is slightly more obvious than in the example above. The component has something to do with the child's behavior.

Kyle is sitting quietly watching "Sesame Street" on TV. His mom is busy baking in the kitchen. The child asks for a drink of juice, but Mother is too occupied to respond. After a few moments, Kyle asks again. Still no response from Mom. Finally, the child raises his voice loudly to be heard. Mom stops what she is doing and gives her son a glass of juice. Later that evening, a very similar situation occurs. The child asks for something but receives no response. Upon screaming loudly, he is given what is requested. Within a few days, Kyle is doing something he had never done before—screaming several times when he doesn't get what he wants.

Analysis: Kyle adapted to his environment. Unintentionally, the environment (Mom) taught the child to scream when he did not receive what was desired. Kyle learned the lesson the environment provided for him. If the environment doesn't change its reactions to the screaming (and to Kyle's asking quietly, nicely, politely), the screaming will adaptively increase and continue.

Behavior	Environment's reaction	Results
Screaming	Mom provides what was requested	Increase in screaming

To discover the previously suggested "additional variable" I asked you to identify, let's first look at the term "behavior pairs." The term will help you distinguish the important "hidden" point, as well as provide a critical first step toward preventing the above undesired results from happening, or changing them if they are presently occurring.

Behavior pairs represent two behaviors. The two behaviors are most often incompatible with one another. That means they generally cannot occur at the same time. (It's tough to ask "nicely" for a drink of juice and "scream" for it simultaneously.) Invariably, one of the behaviors will be viewed as "desired" by a child's parents. The other will be viewed as "undesired." Remember, undesired behavior, no matter how annoying or aggravating, is nevertheless adaptive and purposive. It is the child's way of achieving what he values. Most often, his behavior reflects what his environment has taught him. If we are dissatisfied with his actions, we must teach him alternative ways of behaving. For that to happen, we, most often, must change what we are doing.

Behavior pairs serve as guidelines. They offer structure to both the kids and their parents: the children have a clearer idea of what their parents desire in terms of everyday behaviors, and the parents know the same as well. Thus, they remind us that behaviors occur in pairs—that for every undesired action, there exists a desired counterpart. They help us focus more on the desired things our kids do; they decrease the chances that we will only respond to the undesired actions manifested by the children. With all that in mind, let's find the not-so-hidden additional variable. Kyle's mom will help us.

"Any accidental goofs in the scenario about you and your son?" we ask the woman.

"I gave my son what he wanted when he screamed. That was an error on my part. I should have reacted to him when he asked nicely. The truth is *he did ask nicely*, twice. I just forgot to respond to him. His asking nicely was the hidden variable, right?"

"Yes."

Desired behavior	*Undesired behavior*
Ask nicely	Scream

"The desired behavior was for him to ask nicely. The undesired behavior was for him to scream," she reflects. "Screaming brought him what he wanted. I'll need to watch him and myself more carefully. I'll have to catch him asking nicely and respond to that," the mother says. "His behavior is more important than my cooking."

Where do behavior pairs come from? Parents devise them for their own children. They sit down one quiet evening, look at each other and ask, "What do we want little Billy to do? Do we want him to scream when he doesn't get his way? Do we want him to use a fork when eating? Do we want him to go to bed when requested?" Parents mutually decide on which of their children's behaviors will be viewed as desirable and will represent what the children should do, and which ones will be seen as undesirable, representing what the children would best not do.

Should the behavior pairs be described or written in any particular way? The purpose for the pairs is to provide behavioral guidelines. They should be communicated in such a fashion as to assure that everyone knows what the pairs are telling the children to do. Try this exercise. Which of the following pairs may cause confusion—and why?

Desired behavior	*Undesired behavior*
Be respectful	Be disrespectful
Act maturely	Act immaturely
Not scream	Scream

The first two pairs will create all sorts of problems. Why? Because the terms can represent any number of specific, observable behaviors. In place of the terms "respectful" and "maturely," the parents (and their children) would be better off if the pairs indicated precisely what behaviors the children were to do. In other words, what does a child do when he acts maturely and respectfully? Make sure your answer refers to something you can actually see happen. You want some active behavior, clearly evident to everyone. Now, given the last sentence, do you see anything wrong with the third behavior pair?

Desired behavior	*Undesired behavior*
Not scream	Scream

There is a problem, one that might be fairly serious. Think of the sentence above: You want some active behavior, clearly evident to everyone. Look at the phrase "not scream." That does not tell the child what to do. It only tells him what not to do. Without knowing precisely what to do, a child might inadvertently get himself in more trouble. Try to avoid placing the word "not" in front of the undesired behavior. Try instead to use an active behavior, something the child can do: instead of not scream, try "talk," or "point," or "come get me," or some such active behavior.

Okay, you now have half a dozen behavior pairs listing things you'd like the child to do and to avoid doing. The "to do's" represent behaviors you want to occur often; the "avoid doing's" represent behaviors you'd prefer the child not do. Given that our topic is food-refusing children, your behavior pairs might logically be related to actions associated with eating. If they relate to general activities of daily living as well, this exercise regarding the establishment of clear behavior pairs will benefit the child and you.

What's next? Motivation: helping the child learn to manifest the desired side of the behavior pair while avoiding the undesired side. Motivation brings us back to the earlier issue of environmental feedback. Let's revisit Kyle, his mother, and the determined behavior pairs. This will help us understand how behavior pairs, environmental feedback, and increasing desired behaviors work together. The behavior pairs:

Desired behavior	Undesired behavior
Ask nicely	Scream

Remembering how she initially responded to her son, Kyle's mom now says, "I'm going to give him my attention when he asks nicely. In fact," she says emphatically, "I'm going to give him my attention when he does all of those behaviors listed on the desired side of the behavior pairs. I'm going to catch him doing something good."

Working to Obtain Something Positive

"Catch the kids doing something good." I first heard that statement when I was a graduate student. It's a positive statement. It keeps us, professionals and parents alike, on our toes. It tells us to look for something the kids are doing that fits within our scheme of things and to let them know that we are appreciative of their efforts. Its a "proactive," child-advocacy statement: it means that we are going to help the kids learn by providing them with positive outcomes rather than teaching by only providing negative outcomes or threats of negative things to avoid. We take our behavior pairs; we carefully identify the desired behavior; we watch for it, indeed, help it to occur. And when it does occur, we provide the child with something that she values. "Something she values? A sports car, right?" Somebody's bound to ask that. No, not a sports car. A hug, maybe. A word of thanks, for sure. A sign of appreciation. A word that says that the youngster's behavior has made the day a little easier and a little nicer. Motivation, environmental feedback—with the little kids it's a relative snap. While I've indicated there aren't any certain universal definitions for what is positive and negative feedback, that the individual must decide for herself what does and does not "turn her on," I can't remember one, count them, not one, of all the children I saw that was not influenced, thrilled, elated, joyously renewed, by a smile, a clap, a word of excitement, a warm touch, hug, or squeeze. The kids I worked with all, without exception, wanted and worked for attention from someone (usually Mom and Dad). I was neither Mom nor Dad, but they sure enjoyed even my demonstrative appreciation.

Therefore, take a look at the desired side of your behavior pairs. One may have something to do with eating, like trying a new food, or allowing a spoon to touch a tongue, or sitting in a high chair and smiling, or eating a dime-sized piece of apple. No doubt others will not deal directly with eating, like cooperating when a diaper is changed, taking a bath, going to bed, sharing a toy, asking nicely. Either way, the relationship between the desired side of the behavior pair and positive environmental feedback is simple: catch the kids doing something good and let them know you like what they have done. They will like that; you will like that. Eventually, with practice and fortune, they will begin to do what you want because it pleases them. There's your ideal motivation.

Limits When Necessary

Catching children doing something good and responding to them positively will help them learn to do what you believe is best and important. Diligent as you may be with the above, there still exists the possibility that a young child may acquire behaviors that can begin to interfere with his own growth, development, and eating. First, let me briefly show you how such "undesired" behaviors can come about. Then we'll look at a few ways of dealing with them.

Undesired behaviors can be acquired or maintained in predominantly two ways:

1. *The behavior can bring the child something he values*—Kyle gets his juice after screaming; Kayla gets her toy using the same manner of behavior.
2. *The behavior can enable a child to avoid what he sees as unpleasant, unwanted, or fearful*—Billy protests loudly when it's time for bed, and his bedtime is delayed; Sheila closes her mouth, clenches her teeth, turns her head, and smacks a spoon with her hand as it approaches her mouth, and the feeder places the spoon on the tray and stops feeding.

In both of the above conditions, an undesired behavior, because it has provided the child with what he preferred, will increase in frequency and continue to occur in the future under the same or similar cuing conditions. Again, the behaviors are adaptive and heavy with purpose. The children, by accident, have been taught by their environment (usually Mom and/or Dad) that the behaviors will work. From the children's viewpoint, the behaviors are most appropriate.

When first observing any behavior that you believe may be interfering with a child's progress, it is important to discuss with the other adults in the child's life if they, too, perceive the behavior to be creating some difficulty. Agreement or compromise is essential. If one parent sees a behavior as undesired while the other sees the behavior from an opposite perspective, sparks are going to fly. The child initially will be confused; eventually, he will adapt and begin behaving differently in the presence of the two parents; the different behaviors from the child will likely elicit multiple emotions from the parents that will prevent them from, among other things, experiencing a good night's sleep. However, if the parents reach agreement about the undesirability of the behavior, the next step, a most crucial one, is a mutual decision as to what will serve as an alternatively more acceptable action. With the young child, this step requires a note of caution. Often what we consider to be an alternatively more acceptable, desirable behavior is not at all feasible for a child given his strengths, weaknesses, and general developmental level. Please notice I did not use the child's age in this last sentence. A child's age will not tell us what he is prepared to handle. When considering desired behaviors (academic, emotional, cognitive, or motoric), a child's carefully measured, actively demonstrated, developmental skill level, exclusive of age, is the essential barometer. It is important, therefore, before determining what you might wish the child to do, to check with someone professionally trained to assess the "readiness" skills of the child.

Once a mutual decision is reached regarding what will serve as the desired alternative behavior, you will have developed a behavior pair:

Desired behavior	*Undesired behavior*
Go to bed when requested	Protest when asked to go to bed
Ask for a toy or share a toy	Scream when not receiving what is wanted
Taste food	Push spoon away

The next step is to let the child know that his undesired behavior will not produce a valued outcome. This will require that you watch your actions carefully. You may have to set limits on the child's undesired actions:

1. After a hug, kiss, story, water, Kleenex, etc., bedtime is bedtime, period.
2. A child loses access to a toy for a brief period of time when screaming or refusing to share.
3. You will work through the avoidance responses associated with eating. The turning of the head, the swiping at the spoon, will not prevent the spoon from entering the mouth.

And the final step, the most important one, is to let the child know that his alternatively more acceptable, desired behavior will bring him what he most values—your appreciation, along with the toy if that has entered the scene.

The Diary

You can help yourself and the child with learning desirable behaviors by spending a few minutes watching and writing down how you and everyone significantly associated with the child responds to what he does. Remember, behavior is influenced by the feedback it receives, and often it is much easier to understand the purpose for a behavior (desired or not) by noting the type of feedback the behavior receives. Whenever I am asked to help a child with problems that go beyond food refusal, I nearly always require the parents to do homework for me. While the homework assignment contains several components, two of those components are familiar to you: determining behavior pairs and keeping a diary to see the type of feedback the behaviors within the pairs are receiving.

This record-keeping task need not be laborious. Essentially, it is designed for you and your significant others to see what everyone is doing when the child behaves. Simply write down what the child is doing that is creating some difficulty; note when it is occurring; the conditions under which it is occurring (the cues); how you respond to the behavior; and finally, note the child's reaction to your feedback. Have everyone who comes in contact with the child do the same, and each of you will have a potentially excellent picture of what is happening. You can then begin to see what you all will need to do to help the child acquire alternatively more desired behaviors.

A Child's Sense of Success and Accomplishment

We end this brief sketch on perhaps the most essential of notes: little that I am aware of has a more positive impact on a child than her experienced sense of personal success and accomplishment. Knowing that one can do something and do it well, master it, so-to-speak, no matter how minor or small it may appear to someone else, often provides an unparalleled boost to a feeling of worth and importance. It most assuredly provides the impetus and confidence for trying to master more.

Interestingly, one of the first tasks a youngster is faced with is eating. More often than not, the exercise goes well. More often than not, the child masters the task as though she were unaccustomed to anything else but complete success. On occasion, as we have seen throughout this book, the child runs into a problem—neither of her nor her parents' choosing. Under such conditions, we rally together to find solutions. The task may be difficult; that, too, we have seen throughout the book: children with physiological problems influencing feeding often make remediation arduous. At the same time, the task of helping the child need not be made any more difficult by the acquisition of an undesired noneating behavior that gets in everyone's way. If you are having problems with your child's behavior, run to your diary. See the lessons you and others are teaching the child. Don't allow an errant behavior to interfere with your child's progress. Eating a desired food can go far beyond providing a pleasant sensation to a child's tongue. It can provide the child with a more valuable taste of success and mastery. It can, as Corey's mother implied, help the child realize that she is capable of accomplishing something important. With that comes personal pride, something all of us need.

References

1. For documentation, see *Essentials of Child Development and Personality*, written by Paul H. Mussen, John J. Conger, and Jerome Kagan. The book was published in 1980 by Harper & Row Publishers, New York. The above information is located on page 80.
2. See *Human Development* by Diane E. Papalia and Sally Wendkos Olds. The book was published in 1978 by McGraw-Hill, Inc., New York. The material is located on page 103.
3. Dodson, F. (1970) *How To Parent*. New York: New American Library.

4. Lipsitt, L. P., Kaye, H., and Bosack, J. H. (1966). Enhancement of neonatal sucking through reinforcement. *Journal of Experimental Child Psychology, 4,* 163–168.
5. DeCasper, A., and Fifer, W. (1980). Of human bonding: Newborns prefer their mother's voices. *Science, 208,* 1174–1176.
6. See Judith A. Schickedanz *et al.'s* book *Toward Understanding Children.* It was published in 1982 by Little, Brown & Company, Canada. The material is located on pages 124–125.

Index